# Coping with Vision Loss

# Coping with Vision Loss

## Vision Loss

❖

Understanding the Psychological,
Social, and Spiritual Effects

Cheri Colby Langdell, PhD and
Tim Langdell, PhD

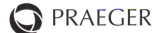 PRAEGER

AN IMPRINT OF ABC-CLIO, LLC
Santa Barbara, California • Denver, Colorado • Oxford, England

**Library of Congress Cataloging-in-Publication Data**

Langdell, Cheri Colby.
    Coping with vision loss : understanding the psychological, social, and spiritual effects / Cheri Colby Langdell and Tim Langdell.
        p. ; cm.
    Includes bibliographical references and index.
        ISBN 978-0-313-34664-4 (alk. paper) — ISBN 978-0-313-34665-1 (eISBN)
    1. Vision disorders—Psychological aspects.    2. Blindness.    3. Medicine in literature.    I. Langdell, Tim.    II. Title.
        [DNLM: 1. Blindness—psychology.    2. Adaptation, Psychological.    3. Medicine in Literature.    4. Spirituality. WW 276]
    RE91.L35    2011
    617.7—dc22        2010041475

ISBN: 978-0-313-34664-4
EISBN: 978-0-313-34665-1

15   14   13   12   11     1   2   3   4   5

This book is also available on the World Wide Web as an eBook.
Visit www.abc-clio.com for details.

Praeger
An Imprint of ABC-CLIO, LLC

ABC-CLIO, LLC
130 Cremona Drive, P.O. Box 1911
Santa Barbara, California 93116-1911

This book is printed on acid-free paper ∞

Manufactured in the United States of America

For Sybil, Melissa, and Alene; Sebastian and Anna; and all our family, together with Eva and Kathy, who greatly inspired and assisted us, and for other friends and colleagues who contributed to this book.

Dedicated to the blind community and to the memory of Mary, Ed, Rudy, and Ted, with love.

"We see by means of something which illumines us,
which we do not see."

–Antonia Porchia, *Voices*

# Contents

# Acknowledgments

For their help and support while we wrote this book, we wish to thank Fernanda and Paul Schmitt and the staff and children of the Blind Children's Center in Los Angeles. We also thank the Reverends Melissa Langdell and Alene Campbell for their interest, assistance, and encouragement while we were writing it. And we thank Annina Arthur for her always brilliant, pertinent suggestions as well as Rahima Nizic-Bonner for her spiritual and moral support. We also thank Kathy McCloskey, Dr. Evangelina de Mirande, and Cecelia Moore, who came to the rescue.

Many thanks, too, to Drs. Ibrahim Jaffe, John Laird, and Randy Nur Hrabko, to Nura and Bill Mansfield, Rahima Wear, Amina Stader-Chan, and other members of the faculty, staff, and student body of the U.S.H.S., particularly to Saida, Hamda, Halima, Rahim, Rahima, Lourdes, and other members of the second year class of 2010–11.

We thank the faculty of National University for their help and brainstorming, and the English Department faculty at the University of California, Riverside, for their intelligent, invaluable suggestions, and for the best literary works on blindness, in particular Professors Steven Axelrod for his help with every aspect of the book and bright ideas, and John Ganim, for his constructive ideas and positive attitude. Gracious thanks, too, to Dr. Diana Glyer of Azusa Pacific University for setting an inspiring example. Warmest thanks go to Diane Williams, Diane Webb, Karen

Herrell, Alice Zimmerman Goetschel, Matthew Rogovein, and Frannie Seamans Collie for their friendship and understanding. To Roxy Han and Dr. Michael Pangelinan, wellsprings of goodness, we offer our gratitude as well.

We thank the Braille Institute's Los Angeles Center for their kind and gracious help.

We thank the librarians at the Young Research Library at the University of California, Los Angeles, and those at the Rivera Library at the University of California, Riverside.

We thank our excellent editor Debbie Carvalko at Praeger for her guidance and her kindness and patience with us, and to Jennifer Boelter, our fine project manager.

Above all, we want to thank Ann Morris Bliss, our wonderful friend, who is the inspiration for this book and an inspiration to us all! Her assistance in research and with every part of the book has better enabled us to write of people's direct experiences and to empathize more fully with the experience of blindness. Without Ann this book never would have been written.

Last we thank the many members of the blind community with whom we have spoken and been in contact: You have helped us immeasurably by sharing your lives and writings with us. We hope this book will give you courage, confidence, inspiration, and strength and that it will answer some of your questions.

Cheri Colby Langdell, PhD, and Tim Langdell, PhD
www.copingwithvisionloss.com

September, 2010
Pasadena, California

# 1

## Introduction

The blind man carries a star on his shoulder
Antonio Porchia, Voices

This book was written for and is dedicated to the visually impaired and blind, and their friends, family, and colleagues who may wish to gain a deeper insight into their condition. In this book we first present one blind person's view of what it is like to be blind, and then we review how blindness has been depicted in world literature. We go on to present a selection of fiction written by or about the blind and then a selection of nonfiction by blind writers. Finally, we present an overview of blindness in the world's religions as well as a brief guide for meditation for blind and visually impaired people, and a chapter on the current state of research on cures for blindness.

### SOME BASIC FACTS ABOUT BLINDNESS

The technical definition of blindness is having visual acuity of 20/200 or worse in the better eye when corrected with lenses. Twenty-one percent of Americans age 65 and over, or 7.3 million people, have some form of vision impairment. According to Research to Prevent Blindness, there are more than 15 million people in the United States with visual impairment, of which 1.3 million people are legally blind. Blindness and visual impairment particularly affect those age 65 or older, and a leading cause in this age group is retinal degeneration.

Worldwide, the World Health Organization reports about 314 million people have visual impairments and around 45 million are legally blind. About 87 percent of the world's visually impaired live in developing countries, and cataracts remain the leading cause of blindness globally. Around 82 percent of all visually impaired people are age 50 or older, representing around 19 percent of the world's population.

## THE FIRSTHAND EXPERIENCE OF BLINDNESS: HAVING THE WHOLE CAKE BUT SMALLER

Possibly no one re-creates the experience of being blind better than the Australian writer, professor, and scholar John M. Hull, who in *On Sight and Insight: A Journey into the World of Blindness* writes movingly about becoming blind, after having suffered from cataracts, as well as a congenital skin condition and asthma. He wasn't fully blind for his first 50 years (Hull 1). His comprehensive philosophical study of the condition and the implications of blindness has a "Foreword" to the blind reader and is an excellent book to read if one is becoming blind. I summarize the most important points here to give a taste of the tone and tenor of his discussions.

Hull's comments in the foreword to this philosophical, phenomenological study are as interesting as they are revealing about what it's like to lose one's sight. He begins by explaining that in 1983, he began keeping a diary both to establish some balance in and control over his life and to record his experiences, dreams, and psychological and emotional responses to his growing blindness. Hull says he started the journal because he wanted to make sense of his life as a blind person and resist any urge he might have initially had to isolate or marginalize himself. He writes it for those with sight and those without so that everyone might understand more clearly and fully how it feels to be blind. He was interested in his own responses to blindness and wanted to observe the changes he experienced in himself throughout the process, to make his life and perspective more comprehensible and thus accessible to his friends and family. In short, he wanted to explain everything novel and different about his new life as a blind man (xi).

This noble purpose—to share the experience of and insights into his own adjustment to the condition of blindness so as to alleviate any distress, confusion, or frustrations others might feel because of ignorance about what a blind person goes through—dovetails precisely with the purpose of this book, which is to educate readers about what to expect when facing blindness. Both we and Hull hope to give our readers insight into blindness in order to make the adjustment as smooth and comfortable as it possibly can be. Hull starts with the following explanation of the process, presenting a viable, positive approach to the experience: blindness does not in principle "lead to the fragmentation of life" (xii).

Losing one's sight does not resemble losing a limb. One is not disabled in quite the same way, and in fact, as we shall show in this book, one need not think of oneself as disabled or challenged at all. The blind person is not constantly conscious of any sense of loss; instead, the personality changes somewhat, but the person is still the same whole person as before. Hull analogized the individual to a cake that has become smaller. The person's life is still wholly integral, the person still himself or herself; it is just that the person's world changes and is more limited spatially (xii). Of course, one still retains the love of friends and family, the love of hobbies and favorite sports: it is just that ability to engage in all the same activities may be somewhat limited and hampered. As driving a car, for instance, becomes impossible, other activities may arise to take driving's place.

The process of integrating body, mind, and spirit takes time, and how long it will take depends on many factors—the person's age at the onset of blindness, attitude toward the experience, and situation in life (xii). Each person's consciousness manages the reintegration of mind and body after blindness differently: "This process of reintegration is piecemeal; sometimes there are moments of dawning realization;...one feels the...gift has been received and assimilated" (xii). At those times, one feels one has understood, opened, and accepted the gift of blindness. So the work of assimilation and psychological, spiritual, and mental integration is not arduous, although it is not a process one can rush. The journey is unique to each individual. And since it is only a process, not a competition, there is no time limit or deadline for the reintegration.

Hull describes his own process of coming to terms with blindness as, first, through understanding it simply as eye trouble, and then later he understood it as a "deprivation of knowledge," knowing that other senses would and could compensate for this deprivation. Then he observed a transformation in his body in relationship to the world and saw that the blind do live in a different world, not different in kind but different in scope from the world of sighted people, a world that is whole in itself and also part of the larger world of those with sight (xii–xiii).

His book is a composite of his observations, forming a mosaic and seeking to understand the condition of the blind from a firsthand perspective (xiii). It affords insight into the new consciousness experienced by a blind person that is brought on by entry into the world of blindness, and it shows how that new consciousness is born. Hull draws together his dreams and hopes, his feelings and experiences: dreams are crucial since one first sees changes in the relationship between the conscious mind and the unconscious mind in dreams (xiii). Next in importance is the "strand of human relationships, since it is in the interaction with others that we know ourselves." These are interactions with friends, colleagues, and most important, his own children (xiii). He has a lot of time to interact with his children and observe how they treat him as a blind person and father. He believes that it is in the study of "the minute particulars" that he has most "grown in understanding" of his condition. And observing the way his children interpret his blindness has greatly affected his own understanding of it (xii). Without the opportunity to interact with them as a father, he would not have developed such a firm grounding in the world and a balanced adjustment to his condition. He then details

> a third strand...[that is] composed of experiences of the natural world. It is the presence of wind, of the rustling leaves of trees, in meditating upon the inexhaustible beauty of the rain, in being awe-struck and terrified by the tumult of the waves on the seashore that I have built up bit by bit the world of blindness. (xiii)

To reimagine and rebuild the world while living with oncoming blindness is quite different in actuality from what one might think it is. Aware of this, Hull asserts,

> At first it seemed as if thunderstorms without any experience of the flashes of lightning could not possibly be as exciting. This was a deficiency-interpretation. As time went by, thunderstorms became not less exciting than before but more so. What the thunder said was heard and interpreted in a new way from the state of blindness. (xiii)

Last, Hull discusses the benefits of his philosophical, theological, and spiritual meditations in his adjustment to blindness. Christian imagery from the Bible was a treasure-house to which he could repair for pictures and stories to embody his life experiences. The Christian tradition drew him like a magnet and offered him both inspiration from the past and a way of integrating his own particular experiences and connecting with a universal dimension in them (xiv). His aims, like ours, are to connect with others—the blind and the sighted—and to reach out a helping hand to other blind people, who, he assures us, are as different from one another as sighted people are. Echoing our impulse here as well, he writes,

> I do not claim to speak for you but only for myself. You...know what blindness is like because you are blind. Perhaps you are reading this book in order to discover companionship with someone else who [is blind]. (xiii)

Hull's is a generous spirit. Clearly he wants to help others, just as we do. His book is packed with insights and observations—everything from his different perceptions as a blind person to anecdotes about how he played and interacted with his toddlers, how he remembered people's faces, how his sense perceptions were altered, and so on.

He was born and grew up in Australia and always had trouble with his eyes, although he did not lose his sight completely until he was about 50. He graduated from Melbourne High School for Boys; at the time, he thought he had a vocation for the Methodist ministry, so he enrolled at the University of Melbourne in 1953, taking an ordinary General Arts degree (5). But just before the end of his first year at university, "the now familiar dark disc reappeared in my right eye." He quickly had surgery and was in the hospital for weeks, teaching himself Braille and reading the Bible (5).

At home as he recuperated, he discovered that his government scholarship would cover a teacher training course, so he studied for one, earning a diploma in education, specializing in religious education (5). And in two years, upon finishing what in contemporary America would be called an associate of arts degree, he was appointed to a position at the Caulfield Church of England boys' grammar school in Melbourne. There he taught English, history, social studies, and religious education, and he coached cricket and soccer (6). It appears he was quite active and useful despite facing blindness.

In 1959 he began his studies at Cambridge University (6). As was the custom in those days, he set sail for England in August 1959 on the SS *Strathmore*; in those days, each American and Australian university student attempted the grand tour of Europe, and early on, through the end of the 1950s anyway, it was customary to sail rather than fly. That was simply more elegant and less jarring than the international flights, which were still in the beginning stages. The goal was to see as much of the world as possible before returning home and putting down roots, possibly never again having the chance to travel.

After seeing the sights of London, he took the train to Cambridge, which he loved. These next years were the most formative years of his life. After long months in the Cambridge University Library and vacations hitchhiking across Europe, he experienced a crisis of faith and realized he could not enter the ministry. He thus determined it would be best to remain in England and pursue a teaching career (6). He also married around this time and accepted a position as a lecturer in divinity in Westhill College of Education in Birmingham, later moving to the University of Birmingham to teach religious education. Eventually, in the mid-1970s, "the forgotten dark shadow made its reappearance" (7) in his right eye, and he went for an examination by a general practitioner, who could find nothing wrong with his eye. But Hull insisted on seeing a specialist, and the problem was diagnosed. He had a quick operation, and his right eye was back to optimal health.

A man born in America less than 20 years after Hull had quite a different experience. Harold Krents, born in the United States in 1944 and blind since birth, describes bitterly in his essay "Darkness at Noon" how he has confronted all the negative assumptions the public makes about the blind: that they can't hear, can't speak, and worst of all can't work or think because they are blind. John Hull seems to have experienced the positive benefits of the condition. If Hull, living in England, tasted the joys of having his four- and then five-year-old son guide him as they walked to school each morning, Krents's essay, which was first published in the *New York Times* in 1976, covers officialdom's negative attitude toward the blind. His essay gives successive examples of the difficult encounters he has while being admitted to a hospital. There, because he is blind, the admitting staff make the assumption that he needs an interpreter, even though he's spoken English since birth. Still, Krents writes, "the toughest misconception of all"—and one that was formerly universal for the blind—"is the view that, because I can't see, I can't work" (235). This particular misconception about the blind is the most injurious to those experiencing blindness or near blindness, since as Krents points out, they are routinely discriminated against in hiring, even when such discrimination breaks federal law. When he applied for positions as a lawyer, Krents received over 40 rejections from law firms, "even though my qualifications included a *cum laude* degree from Harvard College and a good ranking in my Harvard Law School class" (235). When applying for jobs, he was repeatedly told that a blind person could not practice law, "not based on my lack of ability but...on my disability" (235). These rejection letters would today make those firms vulnerable to lawsuits; but in the 1950s through the late 1970s or even into the 1980s, law firms were still reluctant to hire the blind, even though it was illegal to turn down an applicant on the basis of his or her disability. In fact, in the 1950s, a blind Indian child of the upper class such as Ved Mehta was encouraged to study law (*Vedi* passim), at a time when virtually all blind Indian professional men were lawyers. At Pomona College, his advisor asked him, "Didn't you tell me you wanted to become a lawyer or a journalist?" (*Stolen Light* 122). Unfortunately for Krents, however, these experiences became defining moments and were some of "the most disillusioning experiences of my life" (Krents 236). Krents's unpleasant grilling in an Oxford hospital, described in "Darkness at Noon," might not have been because he was blind but because he looked foreign to the admitting officer, who was an older woman. This Englishwoman had met so few Americans or was so provincial that she could not understand American English. On the other hand, Mehta, coming into the American workplace 12 years before Krents, lived mainly in more cosmopolitan or sophisticated places—or possibly Americans are just more open to those who speak English with an accent—and eventually got hired as a staff writer for the *New Yorker* in 1960, when Krents was just finishing high school (Krents 234). Born in Australia and teaching in Britain, Hull, who had not been blind since birth, worked constantly throughout a long and productive career, eventually attaining a high administrative rank at his university, even though he became legally blind around his 50th birthday. His career was crowned by his appointment to dean of his faculty from 1990 to 1994, and he held this role in senior university management successfully, enjoying its challenges.

Hull likens his passage into blindness to a crossing of a barrier or boundary; the passage led to his being able to explore in a more creative way the gifts of hearing and touch" (xii).

On the other hand, he feels that as he leaves sight he is the recipient of grace through his own integrative process in coming to terms with blindness: grace comes as a result of philosophical scrutiny; it "is found in the astonishing powers of the human spirit for healing and rebirth" (xiv).

If the past for this blind man is ringed with challenges that today have disappeared, Hull's success as a blind person in the sighted world and his philosophical scrutiny and theological and spiritual inspiration point the way on the intricate journey a blind person may take toward personal inner freedom.

## COPING WITH LOSS OF VISION

One of the first questions Hull asks in the first entry of his diary, on June 1, 1983, is similar to one often asked of those learning a foreign language: instead of "How long do you have to study a language before you begin to dream in that language?" he asks, "Does the blind person always dream in color or does that gradually stop?" (10). Such thought-provoking questions and their answers form the substance and core of the journal he kept for 12 years, from 1983 to 1991. Although he has been a registered blind person for nearly 3 years, he says that his dreams are still colorful and pictorial (10). Here carrying on with the theme of dream exploration, he asserts that dreams are the best way to decipher the machinations of the psyche. He shows that although individuals might have lost their sight, they still possess the imagination to dream in Technicolor: the spirit and psyche are alive and well, experienced in living color. He comments that his dreams seem to "lag" behind his own psychic reality by six years (13).

In his first years of blindness, he found his psyche began to group the people he knew into two groups:

> There were those with faces and those without faces. It was like wandering around the National Portrait Gallery. Here are rows of portraits, but here is a blank. You can tell where a portrait used to hang by the outline on the wallpaper, and beneath the space is a little label giving the name. The people I knew before I lost my sight have faces but the people I have met since then do not have faces. I used to find the contrast between the two groups of people disturbed me. I could not relate one set to the other set. I knew how I knew the first lot—by their faces. How could I ever feel that I really knew the second lot? (14)

In contrast, a year or so after his son Thomas was born, he had a dream in which he sees his son—looking cheery, robust, a healthy, happy baby— yet Thomas was born 22 days after he lost all sight for good; thus, he'd never seen him. Probably dreams compensate for the images the blind person cannot see. They fill in the blanks, as it were.

Hull notes that he has clear pictures of the people he knew before he went blind but that the pictures in his mind of those he associates with on a day-to-day basis are unclear since either he has never seen them or, if they are children, he remembers a younger version of them (14). He explains that it is because his relationships with everyday people have "continued beyond the loss of sight, so my thoughts about these people are full of the latest developments in our relationships" (14–15). On the other hand, because the relationships with those seldom met or those who are dead remain static or fixed, likewise their portraits are fixed in time. He recaptures the visage of someone he has known in the past by bringing to mind a certain photograph of that person and mentally looking at that

photograph (15).With his wife, Marilyn, and his oldest daughter the opposite began occurring: he slowly began to forget what they looked like,
despite his best efforts to remember them (15). Possibly the everyday presence of his wife is compensation.

Consequently, there is a happy outcome to this predicament—his wife
never ages in his mind: she remains perpetually youthful in his mental
image of her (15). Like the virgins and shepherds in Keats's "Ode to the
Grecian Urn," the spouse of the blind person is fixed in time and never
ages in his or her mind. The loved one is, as Keats writes,

> For ever warm and still to be enjoy'd,
>     For ever panting, and for ever young;
>     And even when the current generation grows old, "Thou shalt
> remain," forever young,
>     "Thou shalt remain." Age can never touch the loved one in the
> blind person's inner eye.

In one season of the television show *Desperate Housewives*, Gabriela,
married to the blind Carlos, spoke highly of the perks of being a blind man's
wife, and other wives and husbands have commented on the comparative
liberation of no longer having their looks judged by their spouses.

This issue of those who do and those who do not have faces in his
memory touches Hull more personally, though. He does remember his
oldest daughter well, based on photographs in his mind, but he has very
few memories of Thomas's face, and none at all for Elizabeth (also called
"Lizzie"), whose portrait is missing from his gallery (15). Of course this is
because she was born after he became totally blind.

Certainly this is a poignant aspect of blindness: to have children and
never be able to see them. Elsewhere, he speaks of how he prides himself
on recognizing Elizabeth when she climbs into his lap and of how his ability to recognize her is very important to them both. So while her portrait
is blank, her space in his heart and mind is filled by his love and knowledge that she is just as much his child as are the older ones whom he saw
before losing his sight completely. Since he can sense and feel her unique
presence, too, she in fact fills the most important place—the place in the
family and in his heart.

Just as sighted people form an image of someone whom they hear every
day on the radio, so the blind too must have a loosely formed idea of how
those with whom they interact look, even though it is unsubstantiated.
Ultimately, Hull states, it makes no difference at all whether or not he
can visualize his three youngest children. While it would be preferable to

be able to see them, he does not think his blindness changes his relationships with them in any way (15). He cherishes them all equally.

Once in a while, he reports, images of people with whom he is talking flash before his consciousness so vividly they are almost like hallucinations. He will see someone, say, smartly dressed, in a pin-striped suit and with a full head of hair (16). This picture may then fade and another may its place, and his colleague may now be portly, balding, missing some teeth, and wearing entirely different attire (16). All these images could become so arresting that dwelling on them could efface present reality; and occasionally he returns to present reality with a start, aware that he's lost the thread of what his companion is trying to tell him. However, he is surprised to observe that he is just as capable as his colleagues at the university in interviewing candidates for positions. While sighted colleagues might be able to comment, for instance, that the candidate's eyes glazed over or that his appearance was untidy, Hull could be picking up on nonverbal cues about the candidate's character constructed entirely from what he heard in the person's voice (17). Hence, in effect, Hull believes his ability to catch nonvisual cues makes up for his inability to make judgments based on seeing faces or clothing.

While he is interested to hear the comments of other men he knows on the looks of a new woman acquaintance, he is most intrigued by the sound of her voice (18). A corollary to this is that, as a result of this process of psychic integration of blindness, he is beginning to lose the category of appearance altogether. He forgets that people do have appearances and has to remind himself of this (19). Having realized that he does not care what others look like, he is then led to wonder what he himself looks like. And of course he is forced to rely on others' comments to form any ideas about what he looks like.

On a lighter note, early in his blindness, Hull was accustomed to greet others with "Nice day!" Yet they might either not respond or be startled and puzzled since they considered that the sort of observation only a sighted person might be able to make (12). But for him the wind has taken the place of the sun in helping discern reality, and he is content with any day when there is a mild breeze, since the wind creates the presence of trees for him. He does not know the trees are there until the wind stirs the leaves. And

> thunder makes [a day] more exciting, because it suddenly gives a sense of space and distance. Thunder puts a roof over my head, a very high, vaulted ceiling of rumbling sound. I realize that I am in a big place, whereas before there was nothing at all. (12)

So what vision does for the sighted person, wind does for the blind: "The sound of the wind in the trees...creates trees; one is surrounded by trees whereas before there was nothing" (12). While the sighted person might comment that a day when the sky is not blue is not a "nice day," Hull would think it is, especially if there is a moderate breeze.

While he can still see a bit, he enjoys taking walks alone (13) along rivers in the Worchestershire and Shropshire countryside and through the Severn Valley. He has to be careful to gauge what is directly in front of him, but he greatly enjoys following the river in his rambles, and these refreshing, successful walks reassure him that he can still manage (13). It is very useful, too, to take a white cane—first a short one, then a middle-length cane, and then the full-size, five-foot-long white cane. He uses it to alert motorists on the road that he is crossing the street (12). This cane gradually becomes essential to his walking.

* * *

Hull notes that because of their inability to see or make eye contact, understandably, blind people sometimes take longer to get to know new acquaintances than sighted people. Not having a mental image of the new person available for reference can sometimes make it hard for the blind to adjust to their new acquaintances and to take them on as friends.

## LIGHT AND DARKNESS: COMFORT AND INSECURITY

Naturally, Hull's children react differently to him because he cannot see. As he "watched" his 16-month-old daughter Lizzie play and twirl with her grandmother, he realized that he would not have been able to experience this if he had been with Lizzie alone, without her grandmother, since she understood he was blind and would not have been showing off to him. Instead, she awaits her grandmother's visit to twirl and dance and show off. This makes him feel consigned to darkness and sadness (20).

This darkness holds a certain disappointment at not having been chosen to witness his daughter's play performance. Conversely, Lizzie's very cheerful presence creates a comfort zone: it pierces the darkness in which he lives, and having her on his knee, while "bouncing her up and down, hearing her laugh, talking with her, knowing everything that is happening to her," he never has "this sense of darkness" (21). The darkness is also dispelled in any environment that is "richly stored with many tactile memories, such as the office and the desk at which I am now working. Every inch of my surroundings, every little object, every piece of paper, every corner or surface is immediately recognizable...known by me" (21). From these familiar objects, he derives a deep sense of security.

He explains that these objects ranged in a certain order afford him pleasure, a kind of spatial and conceptual pleasure (21).

This explanation clarifies the way one achieves a sense of comfort, groundedness, and stability when blind. Familiar objects in expected places, the closeness of loved ones, and familiar spaces all contribute to the blind person's sense of well-being and security and compensate for his or her loss of light.

Generally, too, the degree to which he feels out of place or insecure is the degree to which he experiences darkness. On the other hand,

> While I am engaged in something which gives me a sense of intimate and accurate knowledge, like taking part in a discussion on a subject that I know a lot about, reading an interesting book or making love, the sense of darkness diminishes. (20)

A sense of darkness comes upon him when he feels that he is ignorant of something and has no hope of understanding it or learning how to cope with the situation, as when his little daughter spins and twirls for her sighted grandmother but will not show off these skills for him because it would never occur to her that he could enjoy the performance.

## PLEASE TOUCH

Touch is another element in his connection to the outside world. Since little facial gestures, "the fleeting nuances of the face, and especially the eyes" (14) are lost on the blind person, touch can provide that reassurance and other dimensions of knowing that afford a sense of connection and strengthen the relationship. Since, as Hull implies above, for the blind all the visual dimensions of play do not exist, for them touch and voice make up for visual clues and aspects of play along with much of its spontaneity (14).

Therefore a great deal of subtlety is lost when one loses the visual dimension of communication, yet Hull never ventures into the realm of self-pity. To his credit he never imagines that his condition with its challenges might defeat him. Since he lives constantly in the present moment and finds his close relationships with family members both healing and enlivening, he does not dwell on what he has lost but instead plunges fresh into each new day, realizing that there is nothing to be done about his condition at present.

In another entry, dated July 12, 1983, he writes that touching brings all objects and beings to life for the blind (21). This reflection calls to mind a display of African crafts and baskets called Please Touch, which Hull visited. Such an exhibit would be ideal for the blind person, who cannot count on being able to reach over to stroke the family dog or cat since she or he may not be able to tell exactly where the animal is (unless, of course, the pet is trained to come when called). Hull tells, however, of a welcome time when Thomas was two or three. If he dropped something while Thomas was sitting on his lap, he would lower the child to the floor and let him collect it. Perhaps in the future robots can and will perform this function for all the blind, but certainly, having a toddler playfully pick up what's been dropped is more amusing.

To return to the topic of touch and museums for touch, of course, many museums are not set up for touching. In fact, traditionally, touching has been strictly forbidden in the more august museums in the same way that walking on the grass has been prohibited. Touch gives substance to objects; and touch is what is generally forbidden in a conventional museum. On the contrary, the blind would prefer a museum of touch: in any museum there are plaques that blind people cannot read; and while they might enjoy having a verbal commentary on the museum, they fail to experience the museum itself unless they can touch exhibits, since only touching could ground the descriptions and explanations (21).

On the other hand, a cathedral offers both the excitement of the thunderstorm, in that it affords a blind person a sense of spaciousness, and the tactile dimension museums lack. There is more to touch in a cathedral where, although the person may lack a concept of its architecture in its entirety, still if allowed to trace with fingers its fine carvings and tracery or feel the variety of textures in rougher or smoother areas of stone, the blind person can perceive the physical reality and concept of a piece of art in an exhibit or a cathedral (21). When visiting a cathedral, a blind person does not want to merely walk through it but to run his or her hands over the stone surfaces of steps and floors. Touch conveys the reality of the cathedral better than anything else ever could (21). Similarly, the blind man in Raymond Carver's famous story "Cathedral" does not have the opportunity to examine his cathedral directly, but he experiences it through the drawing he does of it with the narrator while the blind man rests his hand on the narrator's. The experiences of the blind experiencing a cathedral described by Hull and in the short story "Cathedral" are similar: in each case, the sense of touch brings the blind person direct knowledge of the vast and important edifice of the cathedral. The difference, of course, is that in the Carver story the narrator tries to convey this knowledge of vaulted space through drawing the cathedral's architecture with its high ceilings, pillars, and flying buttresses, while from Hull's journals we learn that direct tactile contact with the stone, the screens, the statues, and the carvings produces the satisfaction of direct knowledge and the real sensory experience he craves.

Hull adds that the information gleaned by fingers is not always as accurate or satisfying as sight would be. Even verbal descriptions stop short of giving the whole picture, and he finds it odd that descriptions do not always hit the mark or match what he feels about a person or place. Touch cannot reveal facial expressions that make a face look either ironic or stern or beautiful (21–22). We salute Hull's blunt honesty here: he is frank about what is and is not attainable by or comprehensible to the blind.

## ECHO LOCATION, OR FACIAL VISION

Further on, Hull broaches the subject of that sixth sense some blind persons develop called "facial vision." For him it amounted to an immediate sense of a presence of an object very close to him (22). This vision is a sensory vision upon which some come to depend trustingly, as Ved Mehta did, to the extent that it enabled him to drive a truck around the streets of Pomona as a college student:

> On a dare, I borrowed a Model A truck from Hugh Wire's brother and drove myself from Sixth Street to College Avenue. People were shocked that a blind person should drive a car alone, but there was no traffic on the street, and, with the windows, open, it was almost like riding a bicycle. After all, I grew up around my father's car, and used to drive it a bit in our compound. (*Stolen Light* 362)

First, Mehta learned to ride a bicycle, even seeking to speed ahead of his girlfriend, and then because it was cheap, he buys a car (*Stolen Light* 365) and later drives it on the Pasadena Freeway, with its many twists and turns. Finally a near-miss convinces him and his frightened date that this is madness. So great is his desire to impress his girlfriends and to transcend the limitations of blindness that he goes to absurd lengths to prove, quite logically, that he is as good as any other man since he too drives his own car. Still, eventually even Ved Mehta has to concede that "owning a car will not solve my dating problem, but might alleviate it" (365).

Conversely, Hull explains he might, when attempting to cross a road, suddenly pull back from objects protruding from a truck (22). This extrasensory vision has been a lifesaver for many of the blind, yet it cannot be accounted for logically or rationally, nor can it always be depended upon. Hull says, "This phenomenon is now generally called 'echo location.' It was after the first few months of complete blindness that I became aware of it [but] as long as any sight remained, I was not aware of experiencing echo location" (22). Amazingly, this is broadly similar to the form of radar dolphins and whales use in the ocean to navigate and locate prey, but until now, few understood that the blind used it. It is a fairly well-kept secret. John Hull says he first noticed it just after becoming blind as a student: while walking across his college campus, he became aware of something substantial three to five feet in front of him, and it turned out to be a tree trunk. Going along the path to the university gates, he at any given point knows how many steps he is away from each point on his path toward his destination. He has also learned to perceive the exact distance of trees from him and their relative density or bulkiness. While this mode of perception, available mainly to the totally blind, did not work with thinner objects like a human being or a lamppost, it did alert him to the presence of objects as large and broad as trees (22).

This explains why Ved Mehta did not perceive the presence of a lamppost before he hit it and injured himself—it wasn't bulky enough (*Stolen Light* 265). And perhaps temperamentally John Hull has less to prove to himself and others than the ambitious young Mehta, who at the time was seeking to impress and win over his girlfriend, convinced that he had all his faculties and under the misconception that he was not really blind. Mehta confides in *The Stolen Light*: "(Years later, I realized that almost from the time I lost my eyesight a fiendish fantasy that I could see has remained fixed in my head) (84). And later on in the same novel, Mehta explains his defiant attitude: "After all, I live in the seeing world, and I lead my life as if I could see" (444).

As a more mature adult, Hull has less machismo and possibly more self-awareness than Ved Mehta does, and perhaps we must conclude that the humbler, more positive, and more accepting one is about one's blindness, the easier it may be to cope with it and adjust to it. Still, it is possibly easier on the individual psyche to become blind at 50 when one has had half a lifetime to accustom oneself to the visual world, as Hull has, than at three or four years of age, like Mehta, so Hull has a certain advantage here.

As the months and years go by, Hull feels his sensitivity to objects in front of him growing so that in a short time he "almost never makes contact with a parked car unexpectedly" (22). And gradually he becomes more aware of thinner objects, too. The learning curve is at least in part a function of his awareness and attention to his environment. This explains Ved Mehta's hitting the post: at that moment he was upset with his companions for rushing on ahead without him, paying no attention to him as they hurried to catch the beginning of the film. Hull puts the experience of "knowing" there is something ahead to a perception that he experiences only if he is alone, one that does not kick in if he is "traveling on somebody's elbow" (23). The perception is almost of a physical pressure; and the blind person experiences a sense of presence and a silence, or "stillness in the atmosphere," where before there was empty space (23).

Therefore it is available, almost like intuitive, sensory assistance, to the blind who are alone. Quiet and calm make it more accessible and perceptible. This sense perception, an awareness of presences, is one of the more exciting phenomena in the condition of blindness since it is both unheralded and not widely discussed by the blind themselves or mentioned in literary works. Though literature often assumes and comments on the abilities of the blind to access more knowledge than the sighted can, usually these references are vague and passed over casually. Yet here Hull, a mature professional, a university professor and dean, carefully defines this sense he has of objects he certainly cannot see on solitary walks. What is intriguing is his ability to describe his perception and experience, which he later describes as "essentially acoustic" (23) and "based upon awareness of echoes" (24). Still, he adds, the experience is one of pressure on the skin of the face, hence the original name of "facial vision" (24). The existence of this deeper, almost spiritual dimension in the sensory experience of the blind is positively heartening since there is an implied assistance coming from the universe here—it seems as though one is protected in some sense when one least expects it.

## HOW BLINDNESS AFFECTS THE BRAIN

So much of the information the brain takes in comes from sight; thus, when one loses the sense of sight, the brain, which had been accustomed to orienting itself mainly through vision, experiences this as information loss. Discussing a book by Flo Conway and Jim Spiegelman called *Snapping: America's Epidemic of Sudden Personality Change*, Hull reviews how the authors have accounted for the brain as an organ that needs information to thrive, just as the lungs must have air to breathe. To some extent, blindness can be seen as a mode of sensory deprivation to the brain since much of the information the brain receives comes via the visual cortex (24). Noting that changes in the intensity of the information and in the way it is delivered often bring about personality changes in a sighted person, Hull asks if examining this sensory deprivation in the blind might help us better understand how blindness affects the brain (24). He suggests that we might understand blindness as an event of pure information loss. Some ascribe a sense of drowsiness or boredom and an increase in dreaming to oncoming blindness (25). In fact, Hull states that small inconveniences upset him, like not knowing where he placed his cup of coffee or what he was paid last month (25). When many of these small inconveniences build up, the lack of information can make one uneasy, feel out of control, which is unpleasant for those who are used to controlling their reality.

But he also describes oncoming blindness as a passage from a former self to a new self (25), the birth of a new self, perhaps a more patient, certainly a transformed, self. In another entry, Hull speaks of how much time blind people tend to have to wait for the sighted. Yet conversely, another colleague of Hull's comments to him that Hull is one university professor who never rushes or cuts corners, someone who always finishes every job, and the colleague attributes this to his blindness. Equally, the colleague observes, when he works, he always works right through to the end of a job, never cutting corners the way others tend to do if they can. So these are some of the benefits of the patience and persistence he learns from being blind.

On the other hand, depression visits him from time to time in the first years of his blindness. In the entry "Low Morale," posted on September 22, 1983, he writes that though the progress of total blindness has been so slow as to be nearly imperceptible, writing in his journal has helped him keep track of his loss of vision and its stages. Still, it has been so slow that the moment when he lost the final vestiges of his sight is hard to remember (32). In 1981 he could still see the yellow light that street lamps cast onto the wet footpaths when it rained and he was able to follow the path of the light shining on the road ahead (32–33). By 1983, he can no longer do this, and his morale is at its lowest ebb. He has come to a time when he must realize that his mobility skills cannot improve any more (33), and he must now accept his condition as final and permanent.

At the onset of his blindness, there was a flurry of activity. He was constantly learning new techniques and mobility skills, solving new problems, but now there is never anything left to fear or to lose (33). One respects Hull for not trying to sugarcoat this aspect of the experience and for meeting each thought honestly and head-on. His positive attitude clearly helps him immensely in emotionally, spiritually, psychologically, and physically grappling with his oncoming blindness.

Later on, realizing that one downside of blindness is the passivity it imposes on those who allow themselves to succumb to it, Hull chronicles the ways and reasons he fights depression. The next year, on February 24, 1984, he declares that he feels most frustrated when he is playing with his children (54). Ironically, around those who would probably notice his frustration and depression the least, he feels most frustrated because he feels most powerless. In some sense he wishes they would comprehend his feelings without his having to express them in words. In addition, having been brought up to believe that the father makes the rules, establishes jurisdiction, and gives his children guidance, Hull now feels powerless to perform the fatherly role for his own children.

He is also honest about the times when he feels like a third wheel in his own family: on June 17, in a distorted reflection of Ved Mehta's encounter with the lamppost, Hull is injured while his family crosses the street ahead of him, oblivious to him. Hull calls out, as his family crosses the street, to inquire if anyone is helping Lizzie across. In their intense effort to cross the busy road, though, the family remains silent, seemingly not noticing his question. This upsets him, even though in retrospect he understands that they were merely being prudent in focusing on their crossing at the moment (83). All the same, one can sympathize with a father asking that question and wanting to know the answer, even if it means having to shout a quick reply while helping Lizzie across. No doubt he identifies to some extent with his youngest child, who like Hull himself, was the most vulnerable, the one who needed help crossing roads. He details his emotions at that moment, saying that he feels his fatherly ability to take care of Lizzie has been destroyed, and feels he is a lesser man as a result (83–84).

One wonders why no one—not his wife or the older children— answered him and why they were insensitive to his feelings. Alternatively, a family crossing a busy road *must* be preoccupied with the crossing, especially in Great Britain where the cars can seem to aim at pedestrians, and where it is the pedestrian's responsibility to get out of the way, not the drivers' responsibility to avoid pedestrians. Hull immediately contrasts this experience of feeling useless as a father and protector of his children with his experience of attending a large conference, discussing ideas on a subject he knows well, and making an effort to get acquainted with everyone at the conference, forcing himself out of his passivity. Being presented to new colleagues made the time pass quickly and pleasantly, and he sees that stimulating intellectual work renews and challenges him. Engaged in it, he completely loses any awareness of blindness (84). Hull is fortunate to have had a completely normal academic career, not hampered or curtailed by his blindness. Overall, he is able to discern how his disability has given him special abilities both in interviews of candidates for jobs at his university and in the realm of management.

What he finds most annoying and personally destructive is the unthinking public's infantilizing of the blind person. This may be a phenomenon that existed in Great Britain or America 25 to 30 years ago and not today, but once in a while Hull heard even his friends speak of him as if he were not there. They speak among themselves about where they'll "put" him without reference to him at all, at which point he has to make them aware that they are speaking as if he were absent or were a parcel. This elicits guffaws of laughter (101).

While his friends are jovial and apologetic about this, one can imagine how such behavior might upset a lesser man, and it might be easy for those around a quiet elder or silent blind person to start thinking of and speaking to the person like this.

## SEEING WITH A STICK

Seeing with a white cane is another aspect of blindness Hull accustomed himself to, offering the following more philosophical reflection on this not-so-new way the blind have of seeing and realizing that it must seem bizarre to those who are not blind (33): since the blind person's knowledge is a combination of auditory, sensory, and tactile knowledge, and consequently it is different in kind from the sighted person's knowledge. The blind person sees with a stick.

This is actually quite helpful information, isn't it? It's true that most people are reluctant to step in to help a blind person for reasons indicated elsewhere by Hull: sometimes people ask him if he can manage when he is managing very well, thank you very much, especially if this is his usual walk to work (34). The tone some blind people take can indicate some annoyance at being considered less than competent and thus in need of help. But perhaps Hull is suggesting here that if one sees a person with a white cane marooned or struggling, it is probably best to offer help. Even if the person looks confident, if you see him or her about to plunge into the flow of traffic or in danger, of course it is definitely best to stop that person. Hull himself reports once in a while being saved by observant people who stop him from stepping into unheard, oncoming traffic or from falling into a ditch or from hitting an obstacle he could not detect. Conversely, Ved Mehta refused ever to use a cane since he is adept at walking around open pits and most other obstacles that might have been detected by a cane.

## POTENTIAL AND REAL MISUNDERSTANDINGS

Other misunderstandings between the blind and the sighted can arise when a well-meaning, sighted person tries to help the blind person who walks the same path to work and back every day. One day, a helpful man in the park calls out to Hull that the gate he is approaching is locked; however, a midcourse correction is harder for him to make than it is for a sighted person, since his custom is to walk a certain path and count his steps. He can compute the exact angle of the altered course only if he knows how many steps he is away from the gate; since he can't know that, he must walk to the locked gate and progress to the unlocked gate from there. His would-be helper does not understand this and goes silent. Hull presumes he is shaking his head at the idiocy of the blind man (38).

Such misunderstandings occur even when the blind person is capable and independent, and even so, others try to help him or her. John Hull for the most part doesn't need any help from others unless some unusual hole has opened up in the path or unless there is road work on the route he crosses every day. He counts the steps on each part of every path or road or corridor he goes down, so he virtually always knows exactly where he is. Still, even friends who know him well occasionally want to help him when he needs no extra help: one night a well-meaning friend is dropping him off at home, and Hull asks him to drop him off either just downhill or uphill from his front gate. The friend, thinking he's being helpful in- dicates that, even better, he'll drop him immediately in front of his own gate. Yet Hull comments that this actually puts him in a worse predica- ment because unless he judges the distance exactly, he can miss his gate and would not be sure whether he's gone too far to the left of it or too far to the right. He'd thus be in the embarrassing position of having to fum- ble around, feeling the hedges, and then the friend would feel obliged to get out and help him find his way in (38). Like the prior incident of the locked gate, this is a good example of how sighted people can easily fail to appreciate what it's like to be blind, and what is obvious to a sighted per- son is not necessarily obvious to a blind person.

Clearly it is a matter of pride for independent, highly knowledgeable blind persons to be able to get around on their own without fumbling or getting lost or hurt. While some books for the blind even imply that this can be the plight of the newly blind person, people who have had three or four years to learn how to cope and get around are usually fairly adept at walking normal routes, going along known paths and getting wherever they want to; therefore, they don't want to be helped or interfered with by strangers. Nor do they want others to drop them off at what the driver considers a better place: such misunderstandings occur since the sighted do not always understand the problems the blind face, through no fault of their own, of course. A bit of explanation and dialogue usually solves any problem of blind mobility.

John Hull's musings are often fascinating from a psychological point of view. He is interested in distinguishing between how "blindness affects the process of dreaming, and the way it affects the contents of the dream" (39). Ruminating about this, he wonders how one dreams "about people for whom there is no visual image" and asks whether the blind ordinarily go on dreaming in color (39–40). He asks, but does not always answer, the questions that may occur to anyone who has become blind. He wonders how the blind imagination conjures up a picture of a place the person has never before seen (40). These are questions that psychologists and blind persons have thought about and researched, often with disparate or inconclusive findings.

Probably the funniest misunderstanding in the book occurs at a public conference. Hull was marking time in the foyer, where he was to welcome a prominent speaker and his wife. Hearing a car pull up outside, he knew that the first escort car had pulled up, and the car with the guest speaker would be there soon (193). Hull and his colleagues quickly formed a reception committee and soon he was greeting the distinguished visitor. When the host announced the next guest, the speaker's wife, Hull extended his hand only to discover he'd hit the guest's chin, at which point laughter broke out. The speaker's wife was in a wheelchair, but no one had informed Hull of this. When at last she spoke to let him know where she was, he was able to offer his greetings in the right direction. Upon the distinguished speaker's leaving, Hull found himself shaking the hand of someone other than the speaker, a person who has been seeking to direct him to the distinguished speaker so he could say good-bye to him (193). These small mishaps underscore the need to have a helper for a blind person fulfilling an official role at a formal gathering. Possibly even more important is that the blind person maintain a sense of humor since any lapses in etiquette can be quickly understood and forgiven when the person has a quick wit and is not self-important.

Hull has quite a good sense of humor about his Mr. Magoo–like capers at formal occasions and in everyday life: it's certainly a boon to be able to laugh readily at oneself and at one's own forgivable misunderstandings. Perhaps he would have been better off if someone had taken care to escort and attend to him and perhaps draw his hand in the right direction on this occasion. We can all learn from this incident the importance of having an accompaniment from time to time. All the same, the incident shows the way a blind person's awkwardness can bring out sympathy in everyone around and add to the general jollity of any occasion, especially if, like Hull, the individual doesn't take himself too seriously.

## HOW CHILDREN TEACH AND LEARN FROM THEIR BLIND FATHER

Early on, Hull's children perceived he was different. His situation also elicits his children's sympathy, and Hull uses it to empower his children as they are growing up and teach them leadership. He instills confidence and a sense of competence in Thomas when the child is old enough by letting him lead his father to and from his school. Of course, Hull was always there to protect Thomas, should any danger arise, but Thomas acted as the seeing-eye guide in these expeditions. And from early on Thomas would, for instance, identify a book as his own, as one he could read but his father could not. He would say proudly that this was his book, speaking of himself in the third person; he announced that he could read it but Daddy couldn't. This both amuses Hull and interests him. Thomas would then take pride in reading a book to his father, presumably in order to teach it to him. This entertains them both and surely strengthens his fatherly bond with his youngest children.

On one occasion when Hull puts Lizzie to bed, she is giggling and playful. They engage in a short dialogue about her perception of him and his blindness:

> [S]he said in a teasing voice, "You can't see! Your can't see!"
> "Why can't I see?"
> "'Cos you're a blind man."
> "What's a blind man?"
> Laughing she replied, "It's someone tall and strong and he turns into Banana Man." This last expression was uttered with a shriek of delight.
> Was she just fooling around? Is she associating blindness with other features of Daddy? I do pretend to be Banana Man when I am carrying her on my shoulders down the stairs. Or is she just telling me that I am a pompous old fool and both of us know perfectly well what a blind man is? (140).

She makes the logical point that he cannot see because he's blind. He wonders if she understands the nature of blindness and if she has come to think that all the blind are like her daddy. Could she just be teasing, or is there a grain of truth in her revelry? (149).

While he raises many more questions than he answers, clearly Hull's relationship with his children still flourishes despite his blindness, and his competence at his job remains strong and consistent. Certainly his concern with retaining strong bonds with members of his family and his ability to wonder, observe, and speculate about his state hold a rare appeal for every reader coping with vision loss.

# 2

❖

# A Brief History of Blindness in World Literature

Heart, I said, what a gift it has been
to enter this circle of lovers,
to see beyond seeing itself,
to reach and feel within the breast.

Jalaluddin Rumi

Western literature has long respected the powers and prowess of the blind seer and inspired poet. Homer, the poet of *The Iliad* and *The Odyssey*, embodies the myth of the blind visionary. Although we do not know today if Homer himself was either truly blind or the author of both epics, he is the archetype in Western literature for the blind having special visionary powers and a preternatural understanding, and ability to justify the ways of the gods to men and women. This chapter explores how the public reacts when they see a blind or visually impaired person and the ways the public sees and understands the blind—for instance, the supposition that they have trouble eating because they cannot see the food or the conviction that they are capable of a deeper intimacy with the rest of humanity and have access to the inside story or secret knowledge sighted people cannot attain. We show how the idea of the blind person in society has developed in Western and to some extent in Eastern culture. Mainly looking at works of literature, we examine depictions of blind persons in world literature and show how the image of the blind has progressed and was transformed over the course of two millennia, from Homer's works to *Blindness*, an important contemporary novel by the Nobel Prize–winning novelist José Saramago in the 21st century.

## BLINDNESS IN HOMER AND SOPHOCLES

Like the great Greek playwrights Aeschylus and Sophocles, Homer portrayed blindness, making it significant in his great epics, and he himself was rumored to be blind. He is portrayed as blind in sculpture since being blind is part of his mystique and identity as an epic poet. Most memorably, in *The Odyssey* the aged, almost blind nurse who had raised Odysseus is the first person to recognize him when he returns since she had bathed him before the war and remembers his scar (the dog remembered him, too, and doesn't bark at him as he approaches). Hence one might argue that from the beginning in Western literature the blind have an inside track spiritually and have access to knowledge that others do not have access to through their powers of touch. I don't see this detail as coincidental. Instead, it reveals the more intimate connection many of the blind have or can have with others. They cannot see the surfaces—expressions on faces, flashy clothes, style—so their opinions are not based on superficial characteristics but more grounded in a deeper truth.

Perhaps even more important in the literature of blindness is *Oedipus Rex*, the story of the desperate King Oedipus, who, realizing that he has killed his father and married his mother, in a rage gouges out his eyes so as not to see reality—or so as to see with inner sight and penetrate the spiritual meaning of reality. Oedipus's thoughtless passionate actions embody what the Greeks called *atē*. Defining the Greek word, Jesuit professor Richard Doyle writes,

> ATĒ [which is at the center of Greek tragedy] initially meant "blindness" and in one Homeric passage seems almost to be used in its original meaning of *physical* blindness. At any rate, the evidence for a metaphorical "blindness" is overwhelmingly manifest in Greek epic and archaic lyric poetry, and the meaning does not disappear with the development of tragic poetry in the fifth century. (Doyle 1; emphasis in original)

Thus in the original ancient Greek, the term meant "blind rage." Intolerant, prideful rage implied a blindness that was more a spiritual and mental blindness than a physical blindness. For the Greeks, blindness stems from a spiritual offense against the gods, while in the Bible it connotes physical blindness and an inner inability to see. Then in later Western literature it continues to hold most of these meanings, so in the Western literary tradition blindness has often had both physical and spiritual connotations and symbolic implications.

In Sophocles' *Oedipus Rex,* through the infant Oedipus's rescuers' defiance of the oracle at his birth, Oedipus grows up to carry out his terrible destiny, predicted and ignored. Here blindness represents the power of inner spiritual insight into the truth of human existence and its obeisance to the power of fate. His self-blinding symbolizes a divine revenge wreaked on himself, most terrible because it is self-inflicted. As he puts out his own eyes, his wife, Jocasta, kills herself, exacting divine vengeance on herself. Each must be punished for violating immutable laws they had not previously been aware of. At the end of the play, Oedipus, now a single father, is only just able to be led away grieving by daughters Ismene and Antigone. All of them face a life of pain in expiation for his sins deriving from his tragic flaw. In this and later Greek tragedies, it is not merely "the subjective state of mental 'blindness'" that has determined the tragic hero's fate but also blind "'infatuation,' or 'folly,'" and "the objective state of" blind passion leading to "'ruin,' 'calamity,' or 'disaster'" (Doyle 1). In Homer's epic *The Iliad,* the word never "mean[s] objective disaster.... Always...*ate* is a state of mind—a temporary clouding...of the normal consciousness. It is, in fact, a partial and temporary insanity; and, like all insanity, it is ascribed, not to physiological or psychological causes, but to an external "daemonic" agency'" (quoted in Doyle 7). Hence, from the earliest times, we have blindness embodied in the blind passion born of divine affliction.

Blindness here symbolically opens a window onto the deeper, truer reality, the truth that lies beneath the superficial surface we *think* is all there is of reality. Oedipus is first brought into submission and awareness through his realization of a new meaning in all the major events of his life, and only when he has blinded himself can he see. Hence from its start in Greek epics and tragedies, blindness often leads to a state of spiritual insight and transcendence, the locus of spiritual self-realization. In many texts, from Homer's epics to Shakespeare's *King Lear,* frequently the blind can see truly since they have often experienced suffering leading to spiritual insight.

Like Oedipus, Shakespeare's King Lear, through his blind pride, his tragic flaw, brings on his own ruin and death, and we comprehend too late that mortal humans can perceive the truth only after being chastised by the gods. A character to the plot, Gloucester, is blinded and, only then, realizing his former folly, becomes wise and sees the evils Lear and he have become ensnared in. In Shakespearean tragedy as well as Greek, blindness comes again as a punishment for a hero's hubris, or inordinate pride.

## JOHN MILTON'S "ON HIS BLINDNESS"

John Milton is one of the greatest English poets, and his sonnet "On His Blindness" is probably one of his best-known poems. An accomplished poet in his prime, he has gone blind in midlife. His sonnet considers "how my light is spent" before he can write all that his imagination can conjure up, all the poetry and epics and essays he knows he must:

> When I consider how my light is spent
> Ere half my days in this dark world and wide,
> And that one talent which is death to hide
> Lodg'd with me useless, though my soul more bent
> To serve therewith my Maker, and present
> My true account, lest he returning chide,
> "Doth God exact day-labour, light denied?"
> I fondly ask. But Patience, to prevent
> That murmur, soon replies: "God doth not need
> Either man's work or his own gifts: who best
> Bear his mild yoke, they serve him best. His state
> Is kingly; thousands at his bidding speed
> And post o'er land and ocean without rest:
> They also serve who only stand and wait.

In this famous 17th-century Petrarchan sonnet, the persona, the blind poet, first declares that he has become blind at midlife: "Ere half my days in this dark world and wide" have expired, before he has lived half his life. The one talent he was put on earth to use—his writing ability—the creative talent he could not live without exercising, seems "useless" to him now. This mention of the talent, which "is death to hide," evokes Matthew 25:14–30, the parable of the talents, where the servant who hides his talent meets with death.

So the poem's persona asks, How can a blind man lead a useful life? Can he still serve by writing poetry? How can he exercise his talent? He begins a dialogue with God, asking how he might, though blind, still serve God, his "Maker," and present at the end of life "my true account." Will he be harshly judged if he is less productive because of his blindness? "Doth God exact day-labour, light denied?" In other words, do the blind have to work just the same as everyone else does? "I fondly ask," he says. "Patience" answers that "God doth not need / Either man's work or his own gifts"— our work or human gifts God does not need. But those "who best / Bear his mild yoke, they serve him best." The most obedient serve God best; they bear "his mild yoke." If one follows God's orders, like the other "thousands [who] at his bidding speed / And post o'er land and ocean without rest," one fulfills one's duty to God and is right with God. In the famous last line comes the verdict, God's judgment on this blind poet, the answer to his question: "They also serve who only stand and wait." Take comfort, it says to the blind, if you have to wait to do your work or your accomplishments are delayed. Those who "stand and wait" serve as well as those who like angels "post o'er land and ocean" at His bidding. The race is not necessarily to the swift, as we learned from the fable of the tortoise and the hare, nor are those who seem more efficient and industrious superior to those who have to rely on others to help them do their work. It's well known that Milton depended on his wives and daughters, who read to him and helped him write his poetry from the time he became blind. His final line has been a consolation not only to the blind but also to everyone who is kept from acting by circumstances beyond his or her control. The words "stand and wait" also connote servitude, consistent with the image of the "mild yoke" in lines above. One is a good servant of God if one stands and waits on God's command. True to Puritan theology, one is saved not by works but by God's grace and through obedience to divine command. This redeeming vision of blindness is new in Western literature. Previously, the blind had been conceived of as having been blinded because of sin or by disease; and in ancient times they were thus thought of as rejected by God. Conversely, here Milton claims their membership in the community of the elect and envisions the blind as part of God's plan, worthy members of his royal kingdom: there are those who hurry over land and sea at God's bidding, and there are also "those who stand and wait" for His orders. Milton honors and gives significance to their necessary patience, noting that standing and waiting is noble service, too. At the beginning of the poem, the persona muses that his talent had been "lodg'd" with him "useless"; but Patience, who provides the answer to his questions, assures the speaker that the service of those who wait is also valuable, equally useful, and dignified. Henceforth the blind are given a nobility and spiritual standing in literature as a result of their very being and their waiting on God.[1]

## WILKIE COLLINS'S *POOR MISS FINCH*

Three centuries later, Wilkie Collins, a restrained, proper Victorian novelist best known for his gripping mysteries, wrote a novel featuring a blind heroine called *Poor Miss Finch*, published in 1872. Collins was an especially prolific and popular novelist. One critic explains that his "fictional counter world [was] peopled...by the deviant, the degenerate, and the deranged" and thus it "has enthralled both Victorian and modern readers" (Bachman in Maunder 179). In *Poor Miss Finch*, however, Collins (5) claims to show or "exhibit blindness as it really is," as if blindness were another form of deviance rather than a physical disability. Saying that he has "carefully gathered the information necessary to this purpose from competent authorities of all sorts," Collins asserts in the preface,

> Whenever "Lucilla [Finch]" acts or speaks in these pages, with reference to their blindness, she is doing or saying what persons afflicted as she is have done or said before her. (Collins 5)

So he insists that Lucilla is a typical blind person. But Collins says in the next sentence that his goal is that Lucilla find "her way [in]to their [the readers'] sympathies." The first writers on the blind, wishing to portray the blind positively, occasionally fell into the trap of stereotyping the blind and thereby unconsciously excluding them. In an effort to explore and explain the real life of the blind, Collins reports that he has scrupulously researched the lives of young middle-class blind women and vouches for the accuracy of his portrayal of Lucilla in this tell-all exposé on the blind.

This is not one of Collins's best novels since his characters are unoriginal. Still, it's interesting that this gifted novelist should choose to devote a novel to a blind heroine toward the end of the Victorian era. Apparently his portrayal seemed real enough to his readers: they wrote Collins to ask the address of Miss Finch's eye doctor, Herr Grosse. In his "Note to the Present Edition," Wilkie Collins writes,

> The German oculist—"Herr Grosse"—has impressed himself so strongly as a real personage on the minds of some of my readers afflicted with blindness or suffering from diseases of the eye, that I have received several written applications requesting me to communicate his present address to patients desirous of consulting him! Sincerely appreciating the testimony thus rendered to the truth of this little study of character, I have been obliged to acknowledge to my correspondents—and I may as well repeat it here—that Herr Grosse has no (individual) living prototype. Like the other Persons of the Drama, in this book and in the books which have preceded it, he is drawn from my general observation of humanity. (8)

This fictional Herr Grosse, or "Mr. Big" in English, cures Lucilla. Both characters are highly idealized: she is portrayed as radiant in contrast to others around her, who are, apart from the narrator, often seen as vulgar and dirty or wanting in other virtues or abilities. Herr Grosse is of course dignified and impressive.

When the music teacher who is the narrative consciousness of the book first meets Lucilla, the teacher says to Lucilla, "'Ah, my dear!...I am so glad to see you!' The instant the words passed my lips I could have cut out my tongue for reminding her in that brutal manner that she was blind" (29). But instead of being offended, Lucilla asks, "May I see you in *my* way?" and "held up her pretty white hand," asking, "May I touch your face?" Here we encounter a stereotype found in much later literature—the trope that the blind person cannot meet another person without feeling his or her face with their fingers. The novel continues with a classic scene of the blind woman insisting on touching the visitor's face as a way of knowing her guest. "The soft, rosy tips of her fingers seemed to cover my whole face in an instant. Three separate times she passed her hand rapidly over me, her own face absorbed all the while in breathless attention to what she was about" (29). The blind Lucilla then orders her visitor to "'Speak again!'...I said a few words. She stopped me by a kiss. 'No more!' she exclaimed, joyously. 'Your voice says to my ears what your face says to my fingers. I know I shall like you.'" Hence Lucilla is portrayed as someone who makes her judgments of people based on her feeling of their face and her sense of them through hearing their voice.

Lucilla puts her arm around the music teacher and then instantly withdraws it. When the teacher asks her why, she explains that she doesn't like the color of her dress. When Lucilla inquires what color the dress is, the teacher replies, "Purple." Lucilla replies that in future her teacher must always wear bright colors, never purple, because Lucilla likes to be surrounded by bright, cheerful colors. That she could pick up on a color simply through touch propagates another myth about the blind—that they are clairsentient. Later there are suggestions that she is clairvoyant as well, although certainly Lucilla is not omniscient. Further on in the novel, a gentleman comments that he believes, "you have eyes in the ends of your fingers. Take this, now, and try if you can tell me what it is" (60). Right away she answers that it's a golden vase and asks, "Did you really make this yourself, as well as the box?" (61). And he replies that he has made them both. Later she is also able to describe in detail the pattern on the vase and the birds depicted on it. So she is prescient as well.

Here Collins reinforces most of the stereotypical assumptions and popular myths about the blind. Depicting a blind heroine who is a potential heiress, a person with few family commitments and no profession, he is able to endow her with all the assumed good character traits of the blind. She is shown to have keen perceptual faculties: her very fingertips are able to perceive color as well as intricate patterns. She is refreshingly youthful and displays no false modesty in the presence of a would-be suitor. Her lack of restraint somewhat alarms the narrator, who soon becomes her companion and advisor. Apart from a tendency to be rather childlike, Lucilla lives a comparatively normal, happy life, keen to solve any mysteries in her environment; she is also typically Victorian, eager to attract a suitable husband.

The miraculous healing of Lucilla's cataracts by Herr Grosse is brought in as a plot device to give the novel drama and a surprise twist and is not realistic. The novel's implication that there is a cure for blindness unfortunately misled many readers, who were then inclined to hope against hope that they too could be cured. Wilkie Collins then makes fun of these credulous readers in his note prefacing his next edition (8).

Not Collins's best novel and not really a novel providing profound insight into blindness, *Poor Miss Finch* is still worth noting and even reading because in 1872, the year George Eliot's *Middlemarch* was published too, he purported to write a tell-all novel about the world of the blind, whereas his portrayal of blindness was fairly stereotypical, and he does not shed much light on the world or lives of real blind persons. Still, since the novel unconsciously reflects widespread presuppositions about the blind in the late 19th century, it has value as historical evidence for Western literature's cultural progression in the portrayal of the blind. Later on, many other novelists and writers of all sorts would go on to use blindness as a plot device since it was considered the safest disability to depict in novels, plays, and stories. In most works, blind characters are sadly conventional and predictable. With the exception of the fiction of a few remarkable writers like D. H. Lawrence and Rudyard Kipling, this remained true until the middle of the 20th century and Frederick Knott's play *Wait Until Dark*. This is not the case in Rudyard Kipling's short story "At Twenty-Two," however.

## KIPLING'S "AT TWENTY-TWO"

Published by Rudyard Kipling in 1890, in the book of stories entitled *Indian Tales*, "At Twenty-Two" is a short story in which a blind man stars as the main character. While in *Lazarillo de Tormes*, an early Spanish novel, the main character is a mean old blind man, the main character in this story, Janki Meah, is a wise, yet sometimes harsh, old blind man who is an accomplished miner but not the best husband. He has been blind for 30 years and has realized too late that he should never have married a young "singularly beautiful" (Kipling 84) wife at his age since he has set himself up to be cheated on. He buys her expensive jewelry, "real silver," yet recently she has said that she has never loved him. Instead she loves Kundoo, a younger miner who wants to take her away with him. Behind his back, she flirts "outrageously with Kundoo, and they plan their elopement." Luckily for Janki, he is a manager of a gang of miners:

> Kundoo was really the ganghead, but Janki Meah insisted upon all the work being entered in his own name, and chose the men that he worked with. Custom . . . dictated that Janki, by right of his years, should manage these things and should, also, work despite his blindness. In Indian mines, where they cut into the solid coal with the pick and clear it out from floor to ceiling, he could come to no great harm. (84)

It is significant that according to Indian custom in the late 19th century in the lower castes and classes in India, the blind worked and did ordinary jobs that were considered safe for them, like mining. Janki says, "I have land, and I have sold a great deal of lamp-oil, . . . but I was a fool to marry this child" (85). He has land and lamp oil because he enriched himself illegally at the company's expense, in part at least because the company grants miners no pensions, so they find other ways to provide for their retirement.

Although not all of his gang like him, because he hoards the company's oil illegally and sells it, Janki is revered and respected here because he knows every inch of the mine and remembers everything that has happened in each gallery. Fortunately he knows Twenty-two quite well.

There is a crisis, and Janki and Kundoo are trapped along with many others in Twenty-two. Water is pouring into the mine, and both men and their entire team are in danger of drowning, but Janki is wise and remembers a way out of the top of the mine and orders Kundoo to cut through to the outside. They make it out dramatically, just in the nick of time, amid general rejoicing. All in their gang survive. Emerging from the mine, Janki insists on taking credit for the entire rescue, saying, "Alone I found the way . . . and now will the Company give me a pension?" Immediately he is granted one.

Then Kundoo and Unda, Janki's wife, "steal everything that she could find in Janki's house and run . . . to . . . a land where there were no mines, and every one kept three fat bullocks and a milch-buffalo [a milk-buffalo]" (84). The tone of her speech is headily optimistic: it reflects Unda's inflated dreams of the Land of Milk and Honey she hopes to find in this new place. Here Kipling ironically suggests that their new paradise may not in fact be as pleasant as her former home because Kundoo, who is much younger than Janki, cannot afford to keep her in luxury as Janki had.

The next week, the assistant manager of the mine is talking with cronies, gossiping, and he happens to mention how Janki's wife has run away with Kundoo, and one crony replies, "And those were the cattle that you risked your life to clear out of Twenty-Two!" (91). The assistant manager equivocates, and the story reflects the prejudice and scorn the management, of the upper classes, feels for the miners, of the lower classes, in the pits; even though "the simple pit-folk" believe the assistant manager has godlike powers and none could be killed on his watch, he keeps stoically silent while in their presence and scoffs at them when they are absent. He is well read and refers to Zola's *Germinal*, an important contemporary naturalistic novel, in which a beautiful young girl on the brink of life and her fiancé die in a mining disaster similar to the one they have just weathered. Here the implication is that the crafty Janki may have lost his unfaithful wife, but he got his pension through clever strategizing and stoic endurance. The clear message is that the blind are neither as dumb nor as easy to fool as some may think.


## HELEN KELLER

In the early years of the 20th century, Helen Keller arrived on the scene, a young woman who was brilliant yet blind and deaf after a childhood illness. An innocent American girl from Tuscumbia, Alabama, she is full of sincere concern for others and idealistically expects that others will share her gracious love for all humanity. Perhaps it is not too much of an overstatement to say that she single-handedly transformed the American image of the blind person from ambiguity into an image of someone great, good, even somewhat clairvoyant and clairsentient. Her energetic, positive attitude, her willingness to learn from everyone she met, and her tireless devotion to her great teacher Annie Sullivan impressed all those who knew or met her. Her childlike devotion to her teacher throughout her life was both touching and praiseworthy since many people if they had been helped so dramatically might have gone their separate way after coming to maturity, but Helen Keller wanted to be with and live with Annie Sullivan, whom she called Teacher, all her life.

After Helen Keller graduated from Radcliffe and published her books, *The Story of My Life, The World I Live In, Out of the Dark,* and the famous *Teacher* among them; articles; and essays, the blind population of the United States could no longer be considered less than other people or intellectually challenged in any way. The public was eager to learn of her life and upbringing, since she had overcome the two obstacles of deafness and blindness.

Before the arrival of Annie Sullivan, not even her own family was sure Helen could be a decent or educable girl. Her Aunt Ev saw her intelligence, loved and supported her deeply, and stood up for her in the family battles that decided Helen's fate. Her uncle, Mr. Keller's brother, thought she was animalistic, hardly human, so he thought she should be put into an institution or asylum, while Aunt Ev resisted this on Helen's behalf (Lash 47). Her family was also divided on the subject of the treatment she should receive before Annie's swift success.

Fortunately, Helen's mother had read in Charles Dickens's *American Notes* about Laura Bridgman, a blind and deaf woman at Perkins Institute for the Blind, a school for blind children founded by Dr. Howe (husband of Julia Ward Howe, who wrote "The Battle Hymn of the Republic"); this was the school Annie Sullivan had attended. Laura was about 50 when Annie encountered her; and by then Laura could recognize words and write, but she was still totally dependent on the power of touch in her contact with the world. Inspired by the knowledge that a teacher had helped Laura Bridgman, Annie Sullivan, just 20 years old, came to Helen's home and lived there as part of the family. Within months she was communicating with Helen, who soon sought to learn new words daily and was writing letters by the time she was 7 years old. As most know from the famous play based on Helen Keller's life, *The Miracle Worker*, Annie Sullivan first had to tame the child, since Helen was quite a frustrated, confused child when Sullivan arrived. So Annie Sullivan took her to live with her alone in a cottage near the family home, and she insisted that the child follow her rules and learn obedience. After she became obedient, Helen made unprecedented progress and rapidly learned hundreds of words, which her teacher wrote in her hand. Others noted that she virtually never forgot a word once she had learned it; thus, she was writing in several months' time, and gradually she also learned to speak.

The American novelist Walker Percy called this quantum leap in her education the "Delta Factor," pointing out that it was what made her human: He saw that, before she realized the connection between the water pouring on her hand and the word her teacher was writing in her other hand, "Helen had behaved like a good responding organism. Afterward, she acted like a rejoicing, symbol-mongering human. Before, she was little more than an animal. Afterward, she became wholly human. Within the few hours of the breakthrough and the several hours of exploiting it, Helen had concentrated the few months of the naming phase that most children go through around their second birthday" (quoted in Lash

585). Ernst Cassirer, the German philosopher, commented on Helen's leap in consciousness that he had "discovered with delight that Helen's and Teacher's accounts of the water episode illustrated with astonishing clarity the crucial difference between the physical world of signs and the world of meanings, which he considered to be the distinctively human one" (quoted in Lash 584). While all animals read signs and must read them in order to survive, only human beings connect the world of signs and the world of meanings.

By age 14, Helen Keller was world famous, since news of her miraculous feat—learning to read, write, and speak even though she was deaf and blind—was picked up by journalists, and she became a sensation. Alexander Graham Bell, the inventor of the telephone, whose own wife was deaf, took a special interest in her and encouraged her. A wealthy patron, John Spaulding, also promised to commit funds for her college education—at a time when women were just beginning to attend college—but he died before he could formalize that support system, and other arrangements had to be made. Ultimately Keller did attend Radcliffe, however, and Annie Sullivan sat with her, writing the lectures on her palm, reading to her, and acting as an all-around helper to her. She was the first blind person to graduate from college, let alone graduate Phi Beta Kappa. It pained Helen to know that when she graduated to great acclaim, Annie Sullivan was not offered any praise or credit for the hours she had devoted to Helen's education. Still, Helen sought to rectify that in all the books she published, nearly all of them best sellers. Helen Keller gave Annie Sullivan full credit for her development into a completely mature adult, able to decide for herself her own course in life and to think independently. When her pacifism and political activities later caused many to call Keller a radical, she was vindicated when President Franklin Delano Roosevelt stated that anything Helen Keller was for, he was for (Lash 650). At times during his presidency, Helen Keller was just as famous as FDR, and perhaps at times she was more universally respected than the president.

Throughout her life, Helen charted her own course, pursuing her career of promoting the interests of the blind and of women with Annie at her side, even after Annie married. Helen even became a Suffragette in 1909. Together they traveled the world, supporting worthy causes; they became world famous. To many Americans Helen Keller represented American innocence, freedom, and the ideal of feminine beauty to many who visited her, or saw or heard her speak, or devoured her books. Her deafness and blindness never limited her but helped her reach the masses and speak out on behalf of the blind and half-blind. She wrote extensively about being blind and about growing up blind and deaf, all of which fascinated the

American public. Privileged to meet most of the celebrities of her day and to have a Hollywood film, *Deliverance,* made about their lives in 1919, she and Teacher traveled the world and spoke about their convictions and experiences and in support of education for the blind and deaf. If formerly the blind or deaf had been sent to asylums or institutions for the blind, "put away," as they called it, or relegated to second-class status because of the social stigma, Keller sought to enlighten the public and change all that. Hearing Helen Keller, no one could imagine she was defective, as her uncle had tried to claim initially. In the early 20th century and before, families who had blind or blind and deaf children sometimes hid them away in institutions, thinking there was no way they could be normal and afraid of the social stigma having a "defective" family member would bring on them. While some blindness came about from diseases of the eye, other cases emerged from syphilis, hence blindness was often construed as an indication that at least one parent had venereal disease. Eventually, though, it was discovered that putting silver nitrate drops in a baby's eyes just after birth could prevent infection from gonorrhea; but until then, blindness was either misunderstood as a mark of shame or parents had little knowledge of how to cope with or educate their children since there was no public provision for education for the blind. Keller sought to change all that and worked to get federal funding for the education of blind children and assistance for their families.

While Helen Keller, like Lucilla, touched people's faces when she was getting acquainted with them, she also wrote beautifully of her personal sensory experiences while growing up blind and spoke eloquently, originally, and authentically about her dreams and ideals. Certainly her sensitivity to sensory input informed her clear writing style, Early on, occasionally someone tried to say she was a fraud, but she countered all objections or charges intelligently herself, speaking out confidently and lovingly from heart and intellect about her experiences and ideals. In an America in the midst of, first, World War I and then World War II, she was an inspiration to many and a reminder to the public of American ideals.

Eventually Helen Keller was appointed to the Massachusetts Commission for the Blind and later worked for the American Foundation for the Blind, and she served throughout her lifetime as a spokeswoman and activist for the blind, speaking throughout the world. Working dynamically, she helped get legislation enacted that granted federal funds for reading to the blind and the development of books in Braille. Later in life, she was awarded honorary degrees by Temple University and Harvard University; and in 1953, another film on her life—*The Unconquered*—was released. When she met the young Queen Elizabeth II of England at Buckingham Palace, the Queen told her that Helen had inspired her and given her strength to outlast the German bombings during World War II. Finally, in 1957, about a decade before her death, the play *The Miracle Worker* premiered and spread the word to a new generation of her impressive mastery of language and the written word, and her development into full intellectual maturity, the first deaf-blind person ever to accomplish what she had in the history of humankind.

Strangely, later in Helen's life, with her consent and cooperation, of course, a leading American neurologist, Dr. Frederick Tilney, tested her to see if her other senses were extraordinarily acute by way of compensation for her inability to see or hear. To Helen's displeasure, he found that they weren't exceptional; they were simply "normal, not above average. The results astonished Helen, particularly in regard to smell. She had always been both proud and uneasy over her power of smell, uneasy because a highly developed sense of smell distinguished animals" (Lash 574). In fact, she may indeed have simply been more aware of smell than the ordinarily sighted person and relied more on it than others. Of the olfactory sense, she wrote,

> The sense of smell is the esthetic sense, I think, even more than sight. I know that odors give me a vivid conception of my surroundings. I can smell my landscape because, when I walk or drive through the country, so many odors tell me of fields, streams, honey-sweet valleys and hillsides covered with pines....I am very sensitive to unpleasant odors. They have a depressing influence upon me; for they suggest all manner of dread things—disease, accidents, coming evil and unhappy lives. (quoted in Lash 574)

Her biographer Joseph Lash concludes that even if Helen's sense of smell was not keener than the ordinary person's, she had certainly developed it more fully than the average person does (574). This is because she had to rely on her sense of smell much more heavily than most people do, while sighted people seldom rely on their sense of smell for information about the world since they have eyes to guide them and ears to alert them to possible dangers. Without either eyes to see or ears to hear, Helen Keller used her senses of touch and smell to better effect than the average person.

Reflecting on her extraordinary senses of touch and smell, the paleontologist Loye Miller reported an incident that took place in Pasadena, California, in 1914. He brought Helen to a California maple tree about to leaf and let her smell it. After she felt its buds and branches, to his great surprise she exclaimed that it was a maple even though this was her first trip to California, and of course she had never encountered this type of tree before. Although only half of those who visited him even when the tree was covered in leaves could determine that it was a maple, still she identified it sightless. This experience taught him to use his sense of smell whenever he studied animals or plants. Upon departing, Helen complimented him on the fact that he too used his nose, savoring the smell of whatever he studied (Lash 574–75).

Louise Duffus, Helen's close friend from Westport, Connecticut, described Helen's great enjoyment of the smells of nature, observing that her sense and enjoyment of smell was so great that she could even distinguish the color of the rose—lilac, pink, red, or white— not just that what she smelled was a rose (Lash 575): "Perceptive Helen Keller could distinguish even between the smells of different colored flowers. Is this also in part because of her capacious memory for details?" Today few of us could do what she was capable of, and our age relies even less on smell than hers did. Beyond this, the sense of smell is subjective, and scientific tests are not always accurate or authoritative: Dr. Tilney might have been wrong. Probably Helen Keller greatly relished smell and touch because she had access to fewer senses: thus she made more intense use of the ones she had.

In 1928, though, Tilney, the neurologist, summed up this theory of compensation by pointing out that the phenomena of Laura Bridgman and Helen Keller learning to read, write, and speak show clearly how one area of the brain comes to compensate for "deficiencies in other areas. Helen Keller shows the resultant expansion in understanding and knowledge when the brain is properly importuned to develop them" (quoted in Lash 575). Tilney believed that, with proper training and the use of strategies to enhance the brain's development, the brains of countless others could expand in knowledge and understanding as Keller's did. The only limitation Tilney saw was the inadequacy of instruction and encouragement for the blind: teachers generally lacked the knowledge and skills required to change a deaf-blind child into a Helen Keller. While the brains of blind children usually had the power to achieve what Keller achieved and accomplish what she accomplished, few teachers required their students to develop and improve so greatly.

In that day few had been trained to help those who were deaf-blind: special education as we know it today was in its infancy in the early years of the 20th century. Few teachers knew how to work with deaf-blind children as skillfully as Annie Sullivan had taught Helen Keller, who was quite disappointed in Tilney's conclusions and took them as a personal slight. Still, in the popular press, he was quite complimentary to her and wrote that her "genius will live in the dark world of those who do not see. It will live, too, for those who, though gifted with all their senses, would make the most of their endowments" (quoted in Lash 576). In other words, he knew that Helen's achievements would inspire the blind and other physically challenged people, and they would also inspire and motivate those possessing all their senses to use them more fully and effectively. Helen Keller probably did more than any other person before or since to advance the cause of those with disabilities and to show American society that the deaf-blind are normal persons, not deficient or disabled in any way. At one point she and Annie Sullivan even went on the vaudeville circuit, stopping at nothing to communicate their ideas and their story. Keller shamed those who tried to undercut her or downplay what she had accomplished and impressed everyone with her courage in speaking out on causes relating to the proper care and welfare of the blind and deaf.

### Helen Keller "Sees" the View from the Empire State Building

Often, because Helen Keller's descriptions were such thorough and careful observations, others were incredulous reading them and thought she must have been able to see what she described since she could sometimes portray a landscape better than any sighted writer could. For instance, she was invited to the Empire State Building and upon coming down was asked what she saw:

> Frankly, I was so entranced "seeing," that I did not think about the sight. If there was a subconscious thought of it, it was in the nature of gratitude to God for having given the blind seeing minds. (quoted in Lash 586)

She ends a beautiful description by admitting that probably others saw far more than she did but that she was not jealous of those others. On the contrary, because of her active mind and imagination, she gleaned more information from her observations and thought about what she could perceive more deeply and imaginatively:

> For imagination creates the distances that reach to the end of the world. It is as easy for the imagination to think in stars as in cobblestones. . . .

There was the Hudson—more like the flash of a sword blade than a noble river. The little island of Manhattan, set like a jewel in its nest of rainbow waters, stared up into my face, and the solar system circled about my head! Why, I thought, the sun and stars are suburbs of New York, and I never knew it! I had a sort of wild desire to invest in a bit of real estate on one of the planets....

Let cynics...say what they will about American material-ism....Beneath the surface are poetry, mysticism, and inspiration that the Empire Building somehow symbolizes. In the giant shaft I see a groping toward beauty and spiritual vision. I am one of those who see and yet believe. (quoted in Lash 586)

What have been called her extrasensory insights impressed everyone who read them with her depth of spiritual perception. Her description was published in the *New York Times* and later republished by the president of the Empire State Corporation, Al Smith, former governor of New York (585).

Dr. John H. Finley, the brilliant associate editor of *The New York Times* and President of the New York Association for the Blind, the person who'd written Helen Keller to ask her what she saw from the top of the Empire Building, praised the beauty of her writing and noted that she had probably never thought an ignoble thought, nor had she seen anything unlovely. (quoted in Lash 586)

## D. H. LAWRENCE'S "THE BLIND MAN"

Another famous contemporary of Helen Keller is the novelist D. H. Lawrence, who wrote, along with many famous censored novels, the short stories "England, My England," in which a man is blinded in World War I; "The Rocking Horse Winner"; and "The Blind Man" (1922), one of the first stories written in English devoted solely to a blind man and told from his perspective. The Great War tragically blinded a number of young men, ruining their futures: as it was perceived at the time, blindness was an utter catastrophe, and Lawrence wrote "The Blind Man" in part to reverse the then-prevalent notion that a blind man was totally useless and could not be a complete man but only a cipher. In this story a rich, well-educated, professional male friend visits a young woman, who had been his good friend before her marriage. She is now married; and her husband had been "blinded in Flanders" (430). The average British reader's assumption, reading this in 1922, is that, as she has married him, she must retain a stiff upper lip and stick it out, even though he was considered to be half a man.

The tacit assumption of the narrator seems to be that a blind man may himself feel self-doubt—that he is a lesser man because he cannot see and thus is useless and redundant. Lawrence writes of the blind man, "Sightless, he could still discuss everything...and could do a good deal of work about the place—menial work" (430). The emphasis on menial work at the end is telling: he can no longer, it is presumed, do mental work. The reason why is never explained in the story, so it is difficult to take the leap from blindness to loss of one's mental capacities. Still, the assumption remains, and there is a tone of gloom and foreboding in the opening of the story: perhaps the young wife will fall in love with her urbane friend and want to escape this lonely farm like Emma Bovary. The effeminately named Maurice, the blind man, very much a macho man, seems to worry that his not-very-witty repartee is not sprightly and stimulating enough for her. He is the strong silent type, and he fears he bores her.

The short story begins with his pregnant wife sitting looking out onto a stormy night, awaiting her friend Bertie, who is a barrister, and the stage is set for her to find this new arrival, the witty intellectual man from the city, far more attractive than her slow-talking, slow-moving husband Maurice, who is much more physical than Bertie.

The three eat dinner together, and Maurice leaves the table to do some work. After dinner when Bertie goes to find the husband in his workroom, there is a confrontation between the two men, and Maurice feels Bertie's face in a way that makes Bertie feel physically violated, even humiliated and sickened. The first words out of Maurice's mouth upon touching Bertie are "I thought you were taller" (441), certainly a put-down in modern parlance, but perhaps just a statement of fact 90 years ago when it was written.

Maurice was previously described as "monolithic," and now at the turning point of the story, the crucial moment of their connection as men, he is called "the blind man" rather than by his name, emphasizing the generic quality of this character, possibly indicating that the narrator may not himself take Maurice to be a "whole man" now but just an approximation of a whole man. Bertie agreed to allow his host to touch his face, head, and features even though he doesn't want him to: he endures being touched and even physically examined by Maurice, who stretches "out a strong, naked hand to him" (441). There are sexual implications in the words "strong, naked," as though he is stripping

Bertie naked and overpowering him. Maurice accidentally knocks off his guest's hat. We think this is not accidental. In fact, he wanted to feel his entire head, as we see in the next paragraph:

> Then he laid his hand on Bertie Reid's head, closing the dome of the skull in a soft firm grasp, gathering it, as it were, then shifting his grasp and softly closing again, with a fine, close pressure, till he had covered the skull and the face of the smaller man, tracing the brows, and touching the full, closed eyes, touching the small nose and the nostrils, the rough, short moustache, the mouth, the rather strong chin. The hand of the blind man groped the shoulder, the arm, the hand of the other man. He seemed to take him, in the soft traveling grasp. (441)

The genius of this writing is the way Lawrence explains how Maurice, a sensual man, touches Bertie in a deliberate, but nonthreatening way, "tak[ing] him, in the soft traveling grasp." The use of the word "skull" instead of "head" stresses the elemental, visceral nature of this exercise, and the words "seemed to take him" suggests he is mastering Bertie, overwhelming him, as on a battlefield, or even taking him by surprise. Later, the narrative states that Maurice leaves him "annihilated."

Maurice truly sees through his fingers, and his next observation about "the smaller man," as Bertie is now known, is that Bertie is sickened by this closeness and touch. His brittle intelligence and uptightness make such physical intimacy repulsive to him:

> "You seem young," he said quietly, at last. The lawyer stood almost annihilated, unable to answer.
> "Your head seems tender, as if you were young." Maurice repeated. "So do your hands. Touch my eyes, will you?—touch my scar."
> Now Bertie quivered with revulsion. Yet he was under the power of the blind man, as if hypnotized. He lifted his hand, and laid the fingers on the scar, on the scarred eyes. Maurice suddenly covered them with his own hand, pressed the fingers of the other man upon his disfigured eye-sockets, trembling in every fiber, and rocking slightly, slowly, from side to side. He remained thus for a minute or more, whilst Bertie stood as if in a swoon, unconscious, imprisoned. (441–42)

Like a spider holding its prey, Maurice's grasp and touch keeps the other man "unconscious, imprisoned," against his will. Then just as quickly as he had initiated this intimate embrace, Maurice ends it: "Suddenly Maurice removed the hand of the other man from his brow, and stood holding it in his own. 'Oh, my God,' he said, 'we shall know each other now, shan't we? We shall know each other now.'" (442). Here he seems to be referring to the biblical knowing—a physical, carnal knowing not uncommon among men in Lawrence's day. Obviously this knowing implies an intimacy that frightens and overwhelms the successful professional Bertie. Here is one of the first and raw contests of machismo in English literature, and the blind man, who has won the woman they both love, triumphs over the effete intellectual. Maurice is wholly unaware of Bertie's discomfort, and while the former is jubilant, Bertie is frazzled after this encounter. His only desire is to escape Maurice, who has invaded his space, and the wife sees upon their return that he feels he has been violated by Maurice although the latter does not perceive it.

Lawrence wrote this story to bolster the spirits of the blind—the thousands of war blind men living in England in the immediate post-World War I years when he wrote this story. The point seems to be that even in his blindness—or perhaps because of his blindness, Maurice is capable of "unspeakable intimacy" (432), implying sexual intimacy, shared with his wife. He is capable of satisfying her sexually as Bertie never would have been, had she chosen him instead of Maurice. She and Maurice have bonded deeply and are completely fulfilled, living away from civilization on a farm they both own, which Maurice can run with the help of his staff.

Lawrence probably wrote this story to counteract the false assumption that the blind man is emasculated by his injury and incapable of enjoying a fulfilling life and marriage. For those living the traditional English country life, available to most men returning from World War I (but not to those returning from World War II), blindness does not radically disrupt a person's ability to do work since farm management is more adaptable to the skills and disabilities of the blind: a broader array and variety of skills are called for in farm work, where routine is everything and sight less important.

In this story the blind man Maurice is superior to the professional man physically since he is a Lawrencian real man, fully comfortable in his own skin. The conflict between the two men seems to resonate with a view of blindness that contemporary civilization no longer holds—that the blind may feel useless, redundant, incapable of doing real intellectual work. Lawrence counteracts that false assumption because here Maurice runs the family farm and is a good lifemate for his wife. In fact, there is nothing handicapped about him.

In England in the aftermath of World War I a great many brilliant, promising young men had returned home from the front, having fought as soldiers, and many were ashamed of their disfigurement (Maurice has a disfiguring mark on his face). They were also bitterly ashamed of their blindness because they often assumed they have become parasites on society, men incapable of being independent macho men, or men whom women would not respect, due to their *perceived* disability. In this story, Lawrence successfully counteracts any such impression.

## H. G. WELLS'S "THE KINGDOM OF THE BLIND"

In a vastly dissimilar story, picking up on the idea of the differentness of the blind and their tendency to feel comfortable living with other blind people, H. G. Wells weaves a wicked allegory about sightedness and blindness in "The Country of the Blind" (1938). Wells sets his short story in South America, where a community of blind live in a mythical, remote, nearly impenetrable valley, virtually impossible for the sighted—or anyone else—to enter. Trying to climb a legendary but unreal peak in Ecuador, Parascotopetl, Nunez, the story's intrepid hero, falls down a mountain into the Country of the Blind. Many years before, the inhabitants of the Country of the Blind had been struck by an illness that rendered all their babies blind, so effectively no one in the country is able to see at all. Nunez repeats to himself the famous line "In the country of the blind the one-eyed man is king." He resolves to rule over them all but soon finds he cannot. He is hampered in most of his initial efforts; and, ironically, because he is sighted and in the minority, he labors at a distinct disadvantage because they think he is crazy. They have no concept of what seeing or vision might mean. When he tries to point out to the men and women in the country of the blind that there are other, better ways of doing things, he encounters great resistance and prejudice. No one trusts him or listens to him, and he is scoffed at, belittled. They take him for a fool.

He falls in love with Medina-sarote, the daughter of Yacob, his boss, and asks for her hand in marriage but is refused. He wants to elope with her and waits his chance, but in the early version of the story (1904) he realizes that in order to marry her he must submit to her father's order and have his eyes cut out. On the morning the ghastly operation is to take place, though, he escapes and attempts to climb back over the high mountains to freedom. He becomes ensnared in the mountains and dies. In the later version, published in 1938, the story has a different, happier ending. Here he ultimately escapes with his eyes, his bride, and his life to a country where the sighted are not completely misunderstood. Between

1904 and 1938, 34 years of radical change had transformed England from a country with a traditional monarchy and in which most people adhered to the Catholic or Anglican faith and everyone went to church to a country that was more than half urban and far less traditional or religious. All the old assumptions about class, race, men's and women's roles, professions, and education were being overturned. Change made its incursions everywhere, so Wells wrote about change and its affect on the ordinary person.

A biblical proverb states, "Where there is no vision, the people perish" (Prov. 29:18). Clearly this allegory portrays exactly that scenario and its opposite. The Country of the Blind is the land where the people lack vision, and while the prejudiced blind folk who rule their country may not actually perish at the end of this story, they do not prosper either: because of their wholesale rejection of new ideas, they are left behind by the hero. The blind lead the blind into a ditch. Having sabotaged all Nunez's efforts to show them a better way of life and to explain sight to them, he leaves them behind. The story symbolizes the plight of anyone and everyone who has tried to show others a revolutionary new way of doing something that has traditionally been done only one way. If people repeatedly meet with rejection, they may eventually give up and move away, much to the detriment of those whom they have tried to teach and help. So many aspects of society were changing in the early years of the 20th century when this was written and so many new inventions were appearing that were to revolutionize every aspect of our lives that Wells may have been thinking of any or all of them—the telephone, the automobile, the airplane, indoor plumbing for everyone, not just the rich, electric lighting, and so on—when he wrote this story. Human resistance to change is universal, as this story explains, and those who resist change or deny its benefits may live to regret it. Of course in this story, the blind never learn that they were wrong, and Nunez only barely survives; but the reader takes Wells's point, and one of the most interesting and popular stories of the early 20th century lives on. Here blindness is metaphorical, symbolizing stubborn ignorance, of course, and none of the blind are realistic characters. The story parodies any and all who insist on traditional ways and never give the new a chance but are bigoted, inflexible, and smug, never realizing what they are missing by turning away from innovation and change.

## RICHARD WRIGHT'S *NATIVE SON*

Literary treatment of blindness takes a political turn in Richard Wright's powerful and chilling novel, ironically titled *Native Son*, about the murder of a rich white girl by a poor black boy in Chicago in the late 1930s. *Native Son* (1940) came out just as World War II was breaking out and America was emerging from the Great Depression of the 1930s. Having grown up in extremely hard times in dire straits, Bigger Thomas is forced by relief—the Welfare Office—to take a job as a chauffeur in an affluent white household in Chicago just to feed his family, who have virtually no income. His hard-working, sensible single mother raised him and his brother and sister, who look to him to provide for them since his prospects are better than any of theirs at present; the whole family is largely dependent on Bigger, who dominates his family and kills a foot-long rat in their room in the opening scene but who is intimidated by the white family for whom he will work, the Daltons. Just as the blind man is sexualized in the D. H. Lawrence story "The Bind Man," the black man is also sexualized here. In *Native Son* the black man too lives on the margins of society and is seen as the Other by the black novelist Richard Wright.

Blindness figures in this story both as a reality—Mrs. Dalton is blind—and as a motif. The word *white* occurs quite frequently in the first descriptions of the Daltons and their home: not only do both Mr. and Mrs. Dalton have white hair but they also have a big white cat. Mrs. Dalton is first described thus from Bigger's perspective:

> Then he saw coming slowly toward him a tall, thin, white woman, walking silently, her hands lifted delicately in the air and touching the walls to either side of her. Bigger stepped back to let her pass. Her face and hair were completely white; she seemed to him like a ghost.... Bigger saw that she was old and her gray eyes looked stony. (47–48)

In this encounter, Bigger also learns that Mrs. Dalton has a companion lady who is with her most of the time, but Mrs. Patterson is away and will not be back until Monday. So he is suddenly privy to the knowledge that there are only a few seeing persons in the household. Hence when he later decides to murder the daughter Mary, who he thinks is mocking him, he does so with impunity because the only person around at that time is the blind woman, her mother.

Snow blindness is obliquely referred to here in that seeing all this whiteness makes Bigger feel blind. And when he first visits the Dalton house, Mrs. Dalton thinks it's important that he be introduced to his tasks right away, so he can get the feel of things and "so that he feels free to trust his environment" (48), while Mr. Dalton thinks this would be rushing the process and believes he can be introduced to his duties on another day.

They exchange opinions in front of him, almost as though he were not there: "He felt by the tone of their voices that they were having a difference of opinion about him, but he could not determine what it was about. It made him uneasy, tense, as though there were influences and presences about him which he could feel but not see. He felt strangely blind" (48). His use of the word "blind" here is significant, of course, since it connotes ignorance and limitation. Strangely, although the author Richard Wright is black, throughout the novel the narrative perspective is white, and Bigger is seen as the Other, an outsider, as the sentences above imply.

When Mrs. Dalton prevails and suggests they try to get Bigger started right away, she opens the opportunity for him to begin work on that very day. Even though, sadly and ironically, Mrs. Dalton is as liberal as her daughter Mary, until now Bigger has not realized she is blind, and it dawns on him only when she moves out of the room by guiding herself with her hands trailing the wall: "She's blind! Bigger thought in amazement" (49). The reader might deduce from this that Bigger is either not very bright or so daunted in the presence of the Daltons that he fails to make normal observations because he feels "strangely blind" in their presence. He notices that he is not speaking as much or volunteering as much information as he should be, given this is a job interview. He hates himself for feeling self-conscious and tongue-tied in front of Mr. Dalton: "He wanted to wave his hand and blot out the white man who was making him feel like this. If not that, he wanted to blot himself out" (49–50). He wants to vanish or become invisible—to make them as blind to him as he is to them. Each is blind to the other's reality and consciousness. In the presence of three white adults and a white cat who "contemplated him with large, moist eyes" (51), Bigger is too shy even to raise his eyes to look at Mr. Dalton or to reply properly to his questions. Mr. Dalton, full of bonhomie and humanitarian impulses, asks him whether he'd been accused of stealing tires. But he seems to have decided before Bigger even arrived to hire him no matter what because Mr. Dalton supports the National Association for the Advancement of Colored People (54–55). Bigger, it turns out, has never heard of that organization.

From the start of his employment in the Dalton household, Bigger attributes preternatural abilities to the blind Mrs. Dalton, whom he soon finds alone, standing and listening: she is "in flowing white clothes...standing stock-still in the middle of the kitchen floor....Her face seemed to be capable of hearing in every pore of the skin and listening always to some low voice speaking" (61). He feels she can see him "even though he knew she was blind." The white cat, whose gaze always made him uneasy, was next to her; and at once she detected his presence although he had moved very quietly opening the kitchen door. "Her face was still, tilted, waiting. It reminded him of a dead man's face he had once seen. . . . She knows exactly where I'm standing, he thought" (61).

She questions him about his driving experience and cautions him to be careful. He thinks that "talking to a blind person was like talking to someone whom he himself could scarcely see" (62). What is strange here is that he imagines both that she can really see him because she can sense his presence and hear exactly what he is doing at any given moment, yet he believes this experience of speaking to her is like talking to someone he could hardly see—because she can't see him.

Later that night her ghostly presence in her daughter's room and her calling out for her daughter indirectly lead to his smothering Mary, just to keep her quiet while her mother was checking on her. Ironically, just at the moment Mary gives up her muted struggle and dies, Mrs. Dalton stands with outstretched arms and seems to sense something; she asks if Mary is ill even though she does not seem to be certain her daughter is in the room until she smells liquor and realizes her daughter has been drinking. Her white presence in the daughter's room terrifies Bigger so much that he kills the daughter without realizing exactly what he's done; but afterward he seems to take the fact that he's murdered a white girl in stride, as though it was hardly surprising: he is black, she is white, they were alone together in her bedroom. He believes society will assume that he murdered her, and he will go to the electric chair.

Upon returning home, having disposed of the body by burning it in the Dalton's basement furnace and switching on a fan before he goes to make sure the smell of the burning does not penetrate the family home, he tries to act normal. He even asks his mother for money as he always does, even though he has rolls of money from Mary's purse. His little brother, Buddy, says he would like to get a job like Bigger's; Bigger reflects that although he had not noticed it before, "Buddy, too, was blind. Buddy too was sitting there longing for a job like his. Buddy, too, went round and round in a groove and did not see things" (103). He was trapped in the downward spiral of poverty and did not realize it. Hence Bigger "saw in Buddy a certain stillness, an isolation, a meaninglessness" (103). He does not realize that he himself is experiencing the same isolation and meaninglessness; therefore, he like Mrs. Dalton is blind.

He is aware of his hatred "toward the whites; for he felt that they ruled him, even when they were far away and not thinking of him, ruled him by conditioning him in relations to his own people" (110). He rationalizes the brutal murder as justified in heinous ways aimed at incensing a white audience while at the same time making it clear that the abject poverty under which blacks had been suffering fueled this anger just as the coal fueled the furnace where he had burned the rich white girl. Paradoxically, he sees many other people as blind when he himself is blind to the kindness the Daltons had shown him and the real friendship Mary and Jan, her communist boyfriend, had offered him. Again, the novel indicates that blacks are blind to the reality whites perceive, just as whites are blind to blacks' reality. Bigger is obsessed with ways of getting more power over and money out of the Daltons after the murder, while the family reels in its puzzlement, fear, and worry. Wright suggests that no real communication seems to be possible between the races.

Certainly the image of the blind person here is neither positive nor hopeful but is an image of a person who is lost, one who may have intimations of the truth but who does not quite follow out their implications or argue for what intuition might tell him is true. All of society is blind. After her initial unknowing encounter with the killer in her daughter's room, Mrs. Dalton collapses and withdraws into shocked silence. Bigger's reveries about the blindness of humanity in contemporary civilization continue; and in his racist mentality, when he sees the Daltons again, it is impossible for him to see anything but their whiteness:

> Mr. Dalton's face was dead-white. . . . Bigger saw Mr. Dalton's white hair glisten like molten silver from the pale sheen of the fire. . . . Then suddenly, so suddenly the men gasped, the door behind Mr. Dalton filled with a flowing white presence. It was Mrs. Dalton, her white eyes held wide and stony, her hands lifted sensitively upward toward her lips, the fingers long and white and wide apart. The basement was lit up with the white flash of a dozen silver bulbs. (189)

Just after she appears, the white cat appears as well, following her: it jumps up on Bigger's shoulder, as if to implicate him (since it is the only living creature who had seen him commit the murder), and even when he gets it off, the white cat continues to rub itself against his legs (190). Shortly thereafter, Mary's unburned bones are found in the furnace. Bigger flees and is eventually caught, tried, and killed for his crime. Here it would seem that Wright is not making any comment on blindness but uses the mother's blindness to increase suspense. She was in the room when Mary was murdered, and the plot comes close to suggesting ironically that Mary might not have been murdered, to keep her silent, if her mother had not been there, seeking her.

Sadly, Bigger, who has been effectively silenced himself all his life because of an unjust social and economic system, kills two women—Mary and then later his girlfriend, who works out on her own that he had killed Mary—and he imagines killing many more men and women just to silence them. Accusing others of blindness, he seems the blindest of all since he promotes only his own agenda and wants to satisfy his greed for money, never thinking of the consequences—how much his family will be hurt by his rampage of crime and violence.

## VED MEHTA'S *THE STOLEN LIGHT*

Ved Mehta published an intriguing autobiography, *The Stolen Light* (1989), on the experience of attending Pomona College in Claremont, California, as a blind, or nearly blind, young man from India in the early 1950s. Because of a childhood illness, Ved has been left only with what he calls "my facial vision," which he doesn't explain fully (265). He says he can see nothing at all, but occasionally he seems to have some limited vision. For example, he rides a bicycle and drives a car, both of which imply that he has some vision.

What's remarkable about *The Stolen Light* is that the reader does not realize he is blind for several chapters: he doesn't allude to his blindness or say anything to suggest it for many pages. Only eventually does he confide that he has been blind from four years old, having had meningitis (9). He slips this comment in unobtrusively and deftly, seeking not to call attention to it.

This autobiography, written in the 1980s about campus life in the early 1950s, shows that not only were there no disabled students' services available to blind students then, there was little sensitivity to the blind on campus. Ved has to approach his professor to ask him to announce to the class that he needs a reader to whom he will pay 75¢ per hour. No formal system existed to assist students with special needs, and the professors don't seem to notice he is blind. Fortunately, a student volunteers, and Ved is exhilarated: he had never had anyone read to him for that long. "I felt transfixed, as if I had learned a whole new language in a...day" (95). As he listened to William Faulkner's "The Bear," a complex and symbolic novella, his excitement at discovering Faulkner's rich symbolic world of language grows; the experience was especially intense and significant since he later becomes quite a successful novelist. His reputation is not that of an almost completely blind novelist, however; and in his work he is slow to discuss his blindness, seeking mainly to write about his observations on life and experiences in the world. This has become the trend in current times: the blind professional does not make an issue of his or her blindness but instead enters the professional world seamlessly and naturally, naturally and unpretentiously carrying on daily life and participation in everything required to do the job well. Current technology aiding the blind makes all this possible almost effortlessly. Currently a blind stock broker heads up a major securities firm, and a blind Indian expert in marketing, Sheena S. Iyengar, is a popular professor at Columbia Business School, where she is the inaugural S. T. Lee Professor of Business and the research director at the Jerome A. Chazen Institute of International Business. A ground-breaking researcher, author of many books and articles, she is widely respected in her field. Her short pieces for a mass audience also come out in *Reader's Digest*, and she appears in a variety of media. A film is currently being made about her as well.

Another motif in autobiographies of the blind is the difficulty of eating, and this is one challenge every blind person faces. In his very well-written story about a blind man, "Cathedral," Raymond Carver observes how the blind visitor arranges his food carefully on his plate (Carver 410), so as to know exactly where each specific food is located, and how systemically and efficiently his guest eats. This is a brilliant short story everyone can find easily, by the way, that traces the transformation of a hardened skeptic into a man who believes the blind have much to teach him about the world; it is a story all adults facing blindness should read.

Along with many other stories about his experience of being blind, in his autobiography Ved Mehta describes the difficulties he faces in college while attempting to be served in the cafeteria. Like other solitary blind students, he may occasionally feel that it might be better to forgo food altogether rather than go through the challenges he experiences each night in the dining hall. But he soldiers on, of course, since he must eat, and he finds the other students helpful in getting him into line. Mehta paints such a poignant realistic picture of his plight as a lonely foreign student who was made to feel that anything he wanted was an imposition on other students that it's impossible not to feel sympathy for him. One respects his perseverance in the face of trials others might have buckled under; the reader delights in the humorous ways he describes other students' thoughtlessness and his own sense of being treated like an object— until they come to know him as a person and he becomes a minor campus hero.

In order to earn his scholarship to college, he has already had to suffer through a squab dinner, described in *The Stolen Light* (75–76). There he was *being* vetted by the group considering giving him a scholarship: he is supposed to be intelligent yet also expected to be able to eat the squab deftly. He convinces himself that he had to eat this squab perfectly or he would not get the scholarship. Unfortunately, he was totally *defeated* by the squab. He has to admit that he cannot cut it up and has to yield when someone next to him offers to cut it up for him. Still, his table partner leaves only a few mouthfuls of meat after about 20 minutes of carving. Happily, though, he does get the scholarship anyway, and the reader is left with the knowledge that squab is not the correct choice for a blind person at a dinner.

While similar to his challenges in the college dining room, the challenges Ved faces trying to date are more formidable since they are felt more personally. He is often unable to make casual conversation in social gatherings: "I would sit there envying my easygoing blind-school friend, who, I imagined, would have butted into the conversation of their neighbors, told jokes,...and gradually got people to accept them on their own terms" (96). He was not the life of the party and never could be: he feels the stigma of being blind and does not receive the celebrity reception Helen Keller did. Still, the reader warms to this shy young man who is so often deprived of his milk or salad in the cafeteria (95–96), but who knows what's going on. Until Ved Mehta wrote of his experiences, many blind people suffered in silence, and his is one of the first autobiographies in English about the strange predicaments a blind person faces daily. Hence his books are still good reading for anyone coping with vision loss. He deals with the public's general image of the blind, too: he realizes that the public image of blind people is that they are passive, never taking the initiative (100). So consciously or unconsciously, he sets about disproving that image and showing everyone he is a force to be reckoned with.

Best and most amusing about the book is his recounting of anecdotes of how he takes the initiative and proves to a girl he does not know who suddenly invites him to dinner that he would be a great husband. On their walk to her home, he has already decided he will marry her. Upon meeting her mother, he puts out his hand to shake hers, only to remember that her hands were probably dirty from all the cooking she's been doing; and she immediately reminds him of this, much to his embarrassment. He wants to be friendly and natural, yet is made aware of how important sight is in social interactions.

He had been taught at the blind school in Arkansas not to say that he'd heard a lot about the person he was being introduced to because then the other person wonders what you might have heard, so when the mother utters that phrase, he replies, "Nothing bad, I hope" (102–3). This rather surprises her mother, who asks him to repeat it. Then there is silence, and he hopes that his face "didn't wear the stony expression associated with blind people" (103). In silent frustration he wonders why the girl Anne has left him standing there, not knowing what to do; and the sighted reader can feel his conundrum.

Finally her father rescues him, suggesting that they sit down in the living room, and after a great deal of awkwardness, her father leads him into the living room (104). Then unfortunately Ved and Anne get into a heated argument about whether it is better to become a social worker or nurse or doctor saving lives or to become a writer—Ved's chosen vocation. She argues that saving human lives is a far worthier profession than merely trying to entertain others (104). He retorts by exclaiming that her argument is rubbish and that humans would still be simply animals without art. While he'd hoped for a lighthearted girl who would read to him and help him improve his English and his writing, Anne wanted to be a social worker and save the lives of the great unwashed. He concludes that far from being the cheery carefree girl he'd thought she was, she was depressed (104). Misunderstanding what might in fact have been a true gesture of concern for him in their inviting him for dinner, he now indulges his judgment of her and retreat into sullen silence.

As they walk home in quiet, her hand in his feels "practical and heavy," he thinks (104). He hates being dependent and blind, and he wishes he knew Claremont better and could get himself home, not having to be led (104). He has the degree of self-knowledge necessary to realize that he "was probably no more confused than the young usually are about being dependent and wanting independence, but because of my special situation I was more demanding of others and of myself, and therefore more liable to feel disappointed in others and easily saddened" (104). Hence in this way, he is exactly like other college students, torn between seeking independence and remaining in the comfort zone of the familiar. His transparency is disarming, and his sadness is real and probably universal for the blind. It can truly be frustrating and defeating to be forced to be dependent. Yet the way a person confronts this challenge is the measure of his or her character. Perhaps, as he muses later, Mehta's quarrelsome nature, born of his frustration at being dependent, made him the disabled student the former missionaries didn't invite back, while they would have continued to offer hospitality to a more conventional blind student. In addition, he is not exactly the sort of student missionaries are generally inspired to help since he neither aspired to be a doctor or a pastor, and he is not a Christian. His desire to become either a lawyer or a writer at this point seems secular to them. Besides, although he began the evening thinking he might well marry their daughter Ann, he ends it, bitter and frustrated, certain that he could never love Ann, who isn't a "literary person," but instead wants to be a social worker (104).

In the next chapter he participates in a college tradition, a mud hole struggle, the freshman class versus the sophomores. Someone shouts, not politically correctly, "Get back, you'll get hurt! You blind man, get to the back!" still "[I] managed to squelch forward. I was suddenly in the front rank, raring to go, like a hunting dog that has caught the scent of its prey" (108). Although he is secretly afraid since he is the skinniest man in the fray, he keeps on, struggles with a sophomore, feels he has trounced him, and then is flung off to the side. He greatly enjoys being part of this physical challenge and from then on feels he is part of the campus community. In fact, he is now accepted as a regular feature of campus life, and he comes to know most of the other students and faculty well.

After this, in his own mind he becomes a full-fledged member of the freshman class, not just "you blind man," a generic cripple or, in the parlance of the day, "a handicapped person." This is therefore one of the most important rites of passage of the book since Ved at times seems proud, somewhat sexist and selfish, full of machismo, yet introverted—an unusual combination of qualities for a blind foreigner attending at largely white middle-class college like Pomona in the early 1950s at the high of the cold war. Still, he never alludes to the courage it must have taken to live alone and blind in a strange country, except obliquely in the title of the series of autobiographical books, Continents of Exile.

This is probably the first autobiography of a blind person integrating into "normal" American life, not stuck in blind schools or special schools but studying normally alongside other students. He is able to do it because of his great chutzpah and determination. On the other hand, what is shocking from the modern perspective is the lack of administrative support for his special needs. He is given the college catalog and told to study it, but he has no way to read it. His decision-making process on whether or not to ask his roommate to read it to him is intriguing: he had often considered asking his roommate John to read to him but then changed his mind out of a desire to keep his friendships separate from his business relationships. After all, he had to pay his readers, and he didn't want money to contaminate their relationship (113).

It is sad to think that John is his first sighted friend who is his own age. This distinction between his friends and his readers and paid helpers is no doubt part of every blind person's frustration at being visually impaired. Still, fortunately, he is lucky enough to be able to ask a girl he likes to be his reader. And she accepts that invitation. This small success is offset by the fact that in the prudish early 1950s, before the concept of the teenager came into being, when every college student listened to classical music, and it was thought improper for a girl and a boy to be alone together in a dormitory room, colleges did not necessarily provide any special rooms where blind students could be read to, so he and his woman reader JoAn had to read on the steps of one of the halls.

If steps of buildings or empty classrooms were unavailable, he was forced to read in his own room, having to find times when his roommate was out. One time, however, Ved Mehta is being read to by new reader Gene, and his roommate returns and effectively tells him that he would rather Ved and Gene go elsewhere. Ved isn't confident enough to stand up for himself and insist that, since John normally was not there at that time and Gene and he had started reading before John returned, it would be fair for John to go to the library or go elsewhere to study just for that hour. Ultimately, the friendship between Ved and John breaks down, and they ask for separate rooms. Problems like these arose because he had no place he could use any time he wished unrestrictedly. He even thinks in desperation that he'd probably made a mistake opting for Pomona over the University of California at Berkeley, known as Cal, since as a public university Cal probably had special rooms, even a special library, for blind students; but ultimately he does get a private office in the Honnold Library at Pomona and is the only student with a private office there. Today it seems absurd that there were not services for special students and quaint that the dormitory doors were locked at 10:15 P.M., so students could not go on working in the library after that (137). It was hard enough for sighted students to finish all the assigned work, let alone the blind, who had to make all their own accommodations and who faced untold unforeseen problems like mastering good writing style while dictating. In Ved's case, too, the problem of his perfectionism arose: often he would mull over word choice for hours or days and had to have various versions of sentences available to him so he could choose between them while writing. This might try even the patience of a saint, yet it appears that Miss Rietveld, a patient, very helpful woman he found to type his papers for him, was just that—a saint:

> She was to me like a wailing wall to whom I could go to cry out my struggles with words, cry out my tortured sentences and tortured opinions until I somehow became calm after having them written down on paper. I would leave them for her to type out, and somehow, magically, they would get done. (140)

He asked her not to type while he dictated because it disturbed his concentration while composing; it would seem that he was not the easiest person to work with. On the other hand, his uniqueness on campus must have been traumatic and difficult to accept—unless it was also a point of pride: on September 30, 1952, he wrote, "I am the only handicapped person at Pomona, and the only Indian" (145), and he does not expatiate on how he feels about this.

Along with feeling he is being ostracized because he is blind, he is looked down on because he had very little money and was consequently inadvertently forced to associate with other poorer students. On October 4, he writes in his freshman journal,

> Balboa Island, Newport Beach, Hermosa Beach, Manhattan Beach, Palos Verdes, Malibu. When I asked a fellow who was going to Newport Beach what that was like, he said, "Oh you wouldn't be interested. It's very expensive—you know, a fancy sailing club." (145)

Such disingenuous lack of political correctness reveals the underlying racism and elitism lurking beneath the surface at Pomona College in the 1950s. Thankfully, in the intervening 60 years, federal and state law have been enacted to smooth the way for all special students and to make university study easy by comparison. Still, it is interesting to see the problems that existed and the obstacles Ved faced.

Back then, the goal of every college student was to be popular, and college seems to have been as much a big playground for the children of the middle classes as it was an institution of higher education. At Pomona, Ved has a goal to be a member of the elite group today called resident advisors, then called the Ghosts. He has little hope of being popular enough or getting good enough grades to become a Ghost, he soon realizes; he is automatically excluded, even from freshman hazing activities: on October 18, he complains, "At the Arkansas school, I would have been part of the water-dumping from the Sophomore Arch and tire-pulling and pie-eating.... But here...well, I'm left out. How can I then hope to be a Ghost?" (147). More concerned today about student retention, colleges now would surely not leave a disabled student to cope on his own as Ved was left. Students in the bad old days could discriminate and bully other students cruelly, and many seemed to feel no qualms about silently passing by Ved on college pathways even though they were walking alone, despite the fact that he could recognize anyone he knew by the sound of his or her walk.

By the first of November of his freshman year, he is feeling discouraged, not realizing perhaps that not only have other blind students graduated from college and become successful professionals but that they had been happy at college, so possibly he could be happy, too. Still, Helen Keller at Radcliffe

College had not been left on her own to fend for herself as he was. Instead Teacher accompanied her everywhere, and she might not have tried to be as much a part of mainstream college life as he tried to be. Feeling an outcast, Ved writes that he understands why blind students before him have avoided college, and he realizes that in order to succeed he'll have to work at least "twice as hard" as anyone else, and "keep up my determination and self-confidence, but always appear modest of demeanor, despite my secret vaulting aspirations" (147–48). His secret vaulting ambitions are what drive him to excellence and scholarly success, and these ambitious dreams sustain him in an environment that might have defeated many other students because it seemed a world of tooth and claw if one was blind in the 1950s.

* * *

What emerges from his story is just how normal Ved Mehta is inside—wanting everything that the normal freshman wants, lusting, yearning, hoping for good grades, yet fearing he would fail his courses. He has to resist his urge to put his arm around any girl who is friendly to him and must be aware of the perils of getting a bad reputation. Like any other teenager, his hormones run high: he is a normal 18-year-old boy, so he must control his sexual impulses, though it's extremely difficult. Being independent by nature, he insists that his friends not single him out specially; he dislikes it when students or others try to lead him along (to his mind, leading him like a dog). Yet he scares others by bounding into College Avenue: they fear for his safety. Sadly some other students do not feel they can relax around him and accept him; his sense of isolation is touching, yet not surprising.

Fortunately, on March 6, 1953, "a dinner was held for electing the president of the International Relations Club of Pomona, Claremont's Men's College, and Scripps. Eighty members and guests came…five of us who were running for president were upperclassmen, but I was elected, even though I was freshman, by a two-thirds majority" (163). The reader is relieved that he has finally had a marked success and has found his place in the college. On May 31, he writes,

> It turns out that there are many kindred souls here who I didn't even know existed until I became active in the IRC. These people are not particularly well off. They don't have cars. They tend to be Jewish, or children of missionary parents, and are very serious. (165–66)

Having at last found his own social circle and a group of friends, he finally feels he belongs at Pomona College, and other students across the campus began to accept him, too. Clearly by now, he has also overcome most of the most threatening obstacles in his path and is launched as a full-fledged college student. Every college administrator today should read the first 150 pages of this autobiography since it encapsulates all the woes of being a freshman with special needs. Ved might have experienced the same freshman year of college on any college campus across the country in that decade. Yet his unique story shows both all that can go wrong and all that can go right for a blind student coming from another country and another religion on a college campus. And as Tom Shakespeare has declared, "Because of the widespread segregation of disabled people, many non-disabled people may not have come into contact with disabled people" (quoted in Freedman and Holmes 71). Reading of the isolation, frustrations, and alienation Ved Mehta felt, it is not surprising that 500 miles north in California a few years later Allen Ginsberg wrote of America in his famous poem "Howl," "I saw the best minds of my generation destroyed by madness, starving hysterical naked" (Ellmann and O'Clair 1210–11).

By the end of his freshman year, Ved Mehta had attained a measure of security there. He does apply to transfer to Harvard and is not admitted, however. Over the summer after his freshman year, he chooses to attend summer school at the University of California at Berkeley. There his sexual urges nearly drive him to act overly aggressive with women: "I had but to meet a girl, ... and I would immediately start daydreaming about ... her. Not really as a wife—the idea of a blind Indian man with a sighted American wife was too daunting for me to contemplate—but as someone to touch and hold" (244). Then he meets Mandy, who introduced herself to him in his History in the U.S. class and becomes his reader. He thinks she speaks like a child with a sweet in her mouth until he realizes that in fact she has braces. She is the first girl to speak candidly and openly with him, and she seems much more relaxed around him and more friendly than some of the girls at Pomona. He likes it that she is one of seven children, since he was one of seven, too, as were his mother and his father (250). They attend a play together; he puts his arm around her and expects her to slap him when he tries to kiss her, but instead she kisses him back (251). The next day she resumes her reading to him as before in the noisy section of the library designated for reading to the blind, but finally both confess they are having trouble concentrating. She adds, amusingly, "In my dorm, this place has a terrible reputation. ... Girls say blind boys are always pouncing on them. Blind boys sound so desperate" (252).

Now she becomes Ved's first love; and although he is worried about how she will fit into Indian society, he still wants to marry her. He is as passionate about her as she is about him.

It is not surprising that when he attends Cal people are more tolerant of his condition and accepting of him. Bigger, more cosmopolitan towns may be better places for the blind to live as they may find more services available to them and possibly even more kindred spirits. There they may have access to more advanced technology to assist them and may meet more open-minded people who are more cognizant of their needs and desires.

Finding intimacy is a universal challenge in the lives of the blind—how to form and maintain intimate relationships on an equal basis. To many blind persons, the sighted seem to have all the power. This problem seems to be Mehta's central conflict, and how to meet and resolve it is the central challenge of this book. For this reason, he does not dare confront John, his former roommate and first nonblind friend. Likewise, he supports and defers to Mandy because for the first time he feels like a man, like a gallant suitor, around her. She allows him to help her on and off buses and take the lead when they walk together. But she also helps him find the men's room in a crowded restaurant or anywhere they go (255–57). Initially, as we mentioned before, he had grabbed and kissed her for the first time when saying good night on the steps of her dormitory, expecting to be slapped; but to his surprise she did not. This was a great stride forward for him since he had feared he would never find a girl to love him.

Surprisingly, before Ved ever has his first date, he buys a used car at Pomona College and drives it around campus. For Ved, the act affirms his independence and his ability to take care of himself, while to other students it must have seemed alarming and foolhardy for a blind man to insist on driving himself around. His argument is that there is no one else on the road. His bizarre plan is to find himself a date who would help him drive the car—perhaps steer it with him and navigate for him. During his interview at Harvard, he plunges willfully onto Massachusetts Avenue in Cambridge to prove to the interviewer that he is brave, someone who can take care of himself. However, such behavior tends to have the opposite effect—people are shocked that he is so reckless, and he is not admitted to Harvard. He is trying to find a way to express his originality and creativity, and yet he is not fully aware of the assumptions about the blind at these colleges.

One is drawn to Ved because he is so eager to make his mark in the world, but he has no idea how to go about it. He is assertive, daring, even reckless when he should be polite. Part of his alienation stems from being raised in India and having as yet no clear idea of American manners, customs, or culture since these are not formally taught at school or in college. Without the benefit of visual observations, he is always desperately trying to catch up with others, figure out what's happening. He cannot *see* flirting, for instance, so it does not exist for him. Not to be able to see subtle emotional signs and signals is a daunting prospect, so clearly the blind need more definite and clear explanations, fewer subtle cues. On one such occasion "Mandy unwittingly said something that brought me up short" (258). Once, she came into class announcing that she was wearing a new dress. Although he realizes that she probably only wanted to let him know that she was feeling great in her new dress, he felt bad that he was unable to notice it and compliment her on it. But rather than being grateful to her for telling him, he is defensive and feels inferior because he cannot see and compliment her on the dress.

Self-pity besets him. Rather than celebrating what is good in their relationship, his insecurities make him self-conscious and fearful. On another occasion, they are on a bus, and Mandy begins to speak animatedly with another woman without introducing Ved to her. He hoped she would introduce him, "but she didn't…acknowledge my presence." He wonders why she doesn't bring him into the conversation and thinks, "She's afraid that if she does, her friend will look down on her for going out with a handicapped wog" (259). Of course this incident makes him uncomfortable, especially when Mandy discloses that the woman was her brother Oxford's girlfriend. He is angry, too, but rationalizes this incident on the basis that anyone would be "embarrassed to be seen with me" (259). His low self-esteem, a not uncommon trait in those blind since babyhood, is apparent here. Upon reflection, he later realizes that having her family know about any boyfriend would have embarrassed her, whether or not he was physically challenged since she too was insecure (259).

Another day she asked him if he'd ever considered dating a blind girl: this was the only time she'd referred to his condition (259). She was a very tactful, polite girl who did not want to embarrass or distress him by mentioning it. Unfortunately his reply was not so thoughtful. In fact, by today's standards it could be considered abusive or rude. He calls her question inane, and he tells her he could not consider seeing anyone else since he's with her (259). While the last statement is logical and even flattering, calling her question stupid is offensive. Perhaps this is his revenge for her never offering to take him home to introduce him to her family or even giving him her phone number and address. The rationale he concocts in her defense is telling. He convinces himself that because he comes from such a different country and culture, and their customs are so different, of course she would be ashamed of having him as her boyfriend; thus, living in America made him more and more disdainful of himself and other blind persons (260).

He sounds a bit hypocritical when he says he would discourage his own daughter from going out with a man whom she would have thought of as a handicapped person. In addition, the reflections betray a certain self-hatred, and he realizes that living in the West makes him contemptuous of everything Indian. He compares Mozart's music to sitar music and decides that Indian music comes up short in comparison (260). These statements are alarming since one would expect an Indian to prefer Indian music. In the next decade, the Beatles invasion would hit formerly comparatively quiet college campuses, and Indian music would become very popular toward the end of the 1960s, these shifts anticipating the changes and consciousness-raising American culture and society would soon undergo in the 1970s. His patriarchal assumptions are apparent too in negative musings, and he seems not to be able to make the leap of faith necessary to believe that Mandy might like him for himself. She would disappear for long stretches of time during the day, and he never questioned her about where she went or what she had done for fear of seeming too demanding or needy. He begins to feel their love may not last as long as he'd hoped and begins to get ready for an eventual split (261).

The reader can see how his negative, self-disparaging thoughts undermine the relationship and doom it. Clearly these assumptions that the sighted and the blind truly do not have enough in common to form a lasting bond in marriage make it difficult for him in the sighted world since expectations often create our reality.

Still, Ved has a disarming candor and honesty; he never hesitates to tell the truth, even when it paints him in an less than favorable light. On the last night before the end of the Berkeley summer session, Ved, Mandy, and a group of his friends go to the cinema. They are late for the film and are hurrying—which in itself is ominous. John, a fellow he's recently met, is walking behind the chatty girls; John is awkward when he walks with Ved, and they didn't walk together. So going on alone and trying to prove his independence, Ved bumps into an iron lamppost, badly grazing his head (264–65).

The girls call to the boys behind to encourage them to hurry up, and John shouts that they could just get through before the light changes (265). Then John dashes

> across the street alone. I started to race after him. Suddenly, a truck driver gunned his motor. The noise was so deafening that it completely deadened my facial vision. I veered. I slammed into an iron lamppost so hard that it rang like a bell and sent a vibration all the way down my spine. I have run into many lampposts, but had never before with such a resounding impact. (265)

He has hurt himself enough to stop everyone's progress, and blood is now trickling down from his swelling forehead. He is embarrassed and humiliated, having crashed into the lamppost and once again feels clumsy and inept, singled out by what he calls his handicap. He does not want them to know he has been injured. He's aware he should press his handkerchief against the wound to stop the bleeding.

> But for an instant I felt numb, incapable of the smallest action. I hated John for being inattentive, the truck driver for choosing that moment to drive past. Mandy for not walking at my side—above all, myself, for being handicapped. (265)

To make matters worse, Mandy shouts at him to wait since the light is red, even though she knows he could tell it was red by listening to the sounds of traffic. This call from Mandy destroys their former tacit agreement never to refer to his blindness so as to preserve his self-pride in his autonomy. Together they'd shared the illusion that "I was as mobile as a sighted person," yet this warning shout pierced that illusion and revealed that in fact deep down both of them knew he could never be as mobile as a sighted person, hence he is incensed (266). Blaming everyone else is perhaps natural and understandable under such circumstances. He feels glum as he enters the cinema with the others, crying (266). Mandy shows him some compassion at last, yet he insists on going on in to the film: "We entered the cinema, estranged" (266). This heralds the end of their relationship—his inability to speak openly with her about his feelings at a moment like this.

As one of the blind who have learned to "see with their ears" (so to speak) and attend movies with their friends, not wanting to seem different, he "watches" the film intently, hoping to be scintillating in discussing it later with Mandy and their friends, even as his forehead throbs. Mehta never loses his sense of humor, however; and in the next moment, when he reaches out furtively for Mandy's hand, instead he finds John's and realizes she is sitting on the other side with John between them (266). More embarrassment. If he'd been next to Mandy, she could have kept him aware of what was transpiring in the film: before, they'd developed a way of her cueing him at the changes of scene so as to enable him to stay abreast of the story (267). To his despair, this film was one of those with long stretches of silence; and caught up in what was happening, the others failed to update him. Of course, returning home, everyone was talking about the film, and he was doubly sullen because he had no idea what it had been about. Self-pity and resentment consume him: he tells himself that despite all the obstacles he had overcome or would overcome in future, he would always be just one iron lamppost away from humiliation (267). While his friends, who haven't yet bothered to ask him how he's feeling, engage in a lively debate on what to do with the rest of the evening, he resolves not to continue on with them. When John offers to walk him back to his dorm, he thanks him and says he knows the way and can get there himself. Walking along and hearing someone playing classical music on the violin, he heads toward it to find a group of people waiting outside a closed café where a waitress is now practicing after hours. Rapt, they all listen attentively, and then gradually the others depart until only Ved is left listening. Next he begins pounding on the door of the café hoping she will open up for him, but no one comes to answer the knock. He mulls over the death of his relationship with Mandy and the end of this incredible summer, the summer that at one point he calls the best summer of his entire life.

On his way home, he is now stopped by a policeman, who thinks he's drunk because of the way he's walking: the fact that he doesn't use a cane made his gait resemble that of a drunkard. Learning he is merely blind, the policeman apologizes to him. In this interesting encounter he displays self-possession although he is nearly arrested by the police. Few, though, have the experience of being apologized to by a policeman. He never explains why the policeman thinks he is drunk, but here he reiterates an experience that many disabled persons have since the sighted world does not always immediately perceive that not everyone can see. That does not appear to console him at all, however, and he broods over his loss of face in front of his friends and his own decision not to spend the rest of the evening with them. He must finally face the limits of his ability to sustain the pretense that he is not different from others. In effect, he does not know what to do at this point.

Ved Mehta's burning ambition throughout the book is to achieve what no other blind person in India or America had yet achieved—success in life, in career, and in marriage and family life. But with the prevailing prejudices against the blind in India, he gradually came to believe that he had to live in America, where attitudes toward the blind were much more open and accepting. While his first books tried to some extent to dodge the question of his blindness since he refused to do any special pleading for himself because of his blindness, eventually he saw too that as a writer what he has to offer is his account of his conquering difficulties and achieving these goals as a blind person.

Before he was nominated to Phi Beta Kappa in his junior year at Pomona and was graduated with his class in 1956, he was ask to speak to a group of students about India, and he cast through his archive of former speeches, finding nothing appropriate, but he did write a fine speech chronicling all India's brilliant achievements and how she became free of British rule (*Face to Face* 11). After his speech, a young woman asked if he had ever written anything. When a boy in the back shouted out that writing would be difficult for him, he took that untruth as a challenge. "This challenge, along with that speech, was the germ of the present narrative"—by which he means his first autobiographical volume, *Face to Face*.

*Face to Face* begins with his trying to re-create "a house of India" and the marvelous sights, smells, and colors of the world into which he was born, and then it moves to a description of America as he knew it when he arrives in Arkansas at the age of 15, giving this portion of the book a more personal tone (*Face to Face* 12) There he covers the experience of a boy totally blind, set loose alone in the vast and bustling United States, and the "reception, problems and growth of this blind boy until he reached manhood, and of the pleasures and warm friendships he experienced in the West" (12). These experiences, these problems, these perceptions, and this growth are unique and original to Ved Mehta's autobiographical series *Continents of Exile*. Many people have written about America; few have written so lucidly about discovering the country while blind and at the same time rising to the heights of academic and professional success in courageous defiance of the culture they had been brought up in. Mehta is later hired as a staff writer for the *New Yorker*. In addition, Mehta's novels, all of them, are a delight to read, and they are the source of much detailed information, humorous and otherwise, about cultural attitudes toward blindness; they deflate many assumptions about the blind even as they contradict prejudices and preconceived ideas many hold about the blind in many countries around the world.

## FREDERICK KNOTT'S *WAIT UNTIL DARK*

If many of the works portraying the blind negatively as either helpless, silent, fake, or different, Frederick Knott's *Wait Until Dark* stands in refreshing contrast to prior plays, novels, and films where sometimes the blind are clueless and are only included to create tension, as in *Native Son*. Here the blind protagonist, Susy Hendrix, is left alone by her photographer husband Sam who travels the world. She has recently been blinded in an accident and is getting used to life without sight, when Sam leaves on another trip and thugs arrive hoping to find a doll full of heroin Sam had unwittingly smuggled into the country. They think it's locked in a closet in her home, and the central conflict of the plot is her struggle *not* to give them the key to the closet or release the doll. Until the end of the play, the audience and Susy do not really know if the doll is in the house or not.

The thieves employ various ruses to trick her into giving it up to them—saying they are policemen, for instance—but she remains firm. Sam trains her whenever he is home. He wants her to be truly an independent blind woman—a champion blind woman—and before he leaves they joke about it, but in fact she needs every bit of her training to survive this onslaught of three determined gangsters who stop at nothing. While they have an array of powerful weapons and psychological strategies to terrify her, she has in her arsenal only darkness; kitchen knives, which she hides in her sleeve; and her firm resolve not to be intimidated. In a final skirmish with the last killer to bully her—the rest are already dead—Susy meets her assailant in what she hopes is pitch darkness and after a struggle prevails and kills him. When the police come, she is still cowering terrified behind the refrigerator, and it's several minutes before one lights a match and sees her. A little girl, Gloria, who had taken the doll home with her to play with, assures her that she will be all right and leads her off to comfort her while the police deal with the bodies. In the film version, which aims to resemble the end of *Breakfast at Tiffany's*, she is reunited with her husband and the little girl, who is the only person who has been helping her in this ordeal.

Here the blind leading lady is courageous, firm, and strong until she finally shows fear in the last act of the play: she acts contrary to the stereotype since she is everything one does not expect a blind woman to be—resourceful, independent, brave in the face of unrelenting intimidation. Even when the criminals who have broken into her Greenwich Village flat say that her husband is wanted by the police and they are trying to help him and that she'd be helping him out if she relinquished the doll, she refuses to relent. Debuting in the late 1960s and concurrent with the student riots that closed down many American college campuses, this might be called a feminist play since it catches the fighting spirit of the times and heralds the women's movement that was getting under way in 1967 and growing in the early 1970s. Susy is, above all, a woman of native nobility who holds her own against men with criminal or base intent. Her husband, Sam, in leaving her alone, seems somewhat insensitive to her personal plight, yet much worse is the later onslaught of thugs in search of the doll. This very positive portrayal of a blind woman, later expertly acted by Audrey Hepburn in the film, fuels the suspense since the audience increasingly identifies with her and fears she will be killed as the mob threats become more and more frightening and she moves from firmness to eventual terror herself. Still, this image of the blind woman as heroine is new and unique to literature, and one we hope to see more of. The play had quite a successful year-long run on Broadway and was even more successful in London, where the setting was changed to Notting Hill.

## JAMES KELMAN

Scotsman James Kelman covers another aspect of being human—one we have not yet touched on so far—in an original, sometimes humorous stream-of-consciousness millennial novel set in downtown Glasgow. He sets the tone for his outrageous howl of a novel about another side of the experience of being blind, destitute, on the streets, and mostly homeless in the first sentence of *How Late It Was, How Late* (1994):

> Ye wake in a corner and stay there hoping your body will disappear, the thoughts smoldering ye; these thoughts; but ye want to remember and face up to things, just something keeps ye from doing it, what can ye no do it; the words filling your head: then the other words, there's something wrong, there's something far wrong.... Edging back into awareness of where ye are: here, slumped in this corner, with these thoughts filling ye. And oh Christ his back was sore; still and the head pounding. He shivered and hunched up his shoulders, shut his eyes, rubbed into the corners with his fingertips; seeing all kinds of spots and lights. (1)

The Scots dialect, frequent expletives, and misery reflect the actual experience of trying to survive on the mean streets of Glasgow. The mean streets are the home and environment of this Glaswegian ex-con Sammy, who peppers each page with the f-word. This novel won the Booker Prize the year it was published, shocking the British literary establishment. Its hero had been criticized as being weak and slow to work out any of his problems, yet constantly obsessed by them, and the characterizations could be called indistinct.

Sammy, the narrator, instigates a fight with and is throttled by soldiers. When he regains consciousness he is blind. So in some sense he has blinded himself for reasons that are not ever made clear, and his life then revolves around dealing with "the DSS Central Medical" facility (224); trying to get treatment and help, which seldom comes; his dealings with women, especially his girlfriend Helen; avoiding getting his clothes and belongings stolen; and simply staying alive. The medical authorities are not even convinced he's really blind, which enrages him, and he calls them idiots and swears at them, which of course doesn't help his situation.

Now and then he is aided by some—handed onto buses, given medical help—but his world remains desperate, confused, so here the world of the blind is portrayed with forthright realism and gutter frankness.

His musings, here and there eloquent and elsewhere repetitive ravings, treat on the general blindness of the human condition and the way we must work out our problems individually if and when we find ourselves homeless, alone, and broke on the cold streets of Glasgow, the grittiest metropolitan center in Scotland. Some have compared Sammy to a character of Samuel Beckett or Albert Camus. Because he blinds himself, though less consciously than Oedipus, the novel has been compared to *Oedipus Rex*. Still, it is too rambling and too full of profanity to suit many readers. Gradually, as the reader comes to know him, we may feel compassion for Sammy, yet wonder at the extent of his problems. But it may also be human nature not to sympathize at first with people who have such vastly different lives and lifestyles than ourselves, and maybe that is Kelman's point—to show us that, denied state or government help, the blind can become destitute. There is always a hint that Sammy has a psychosis or neurosis that further hinders him from living as well and independently as he might, yet he also vehemently denies this and refuses psychological help or treatment. The ambiguities are many here, but the novel is like an intricate puzzle that rewards careful reading.

## DAVID WHYTE'S "SWEET DARKNESS"

Spiritual progress or spiritual standing is unaffected by ability to see with one's physical eyes. When it comes to enlightenment in any of the religious traditions, physical sight is far less important than one's inner sight or divine insight. David Whyte develops this idea in his superb poem "Sweet Darkness": "When your vision has gone / no part of the world can find you." Hence for the one experiencing this loss of outer vision and strengthening of inner vision and insight, it is now "time to go into the dark / When the night has eyes / to recognize its own." To move into sweet darkness, "you can be sure / you are not beyond love." The "you" to whom the poem is addressed is assured "the dark will be your womb / tonight." And "the night will give you a horizon / further than you can see." And the reader, now basking in luxuriant darkness, the womb of the night, is told, "You must learn one thing: / the world was made to be free in." And clearly the listener is invited to enjoy that freedom here and now and to "give up all the other worlds / except the one to which you belong" because "sometimes it takes darkness and the sweet / confinement of your aloneness to learn" that "anything or anyone / that does not bring you alive / is too small for you." Here the poem moves the reader from loss of outward sight to luxuriance in and deep enjoyment of life. The point of life is to enjoy it, to be free in the vastness of space and to know that whatever does not "bring you alive" is "too small for you." Whatever cramps, limits, or constrains you is not worth your time and effort; it is nothing to worry about. Your purpose on earth is to enjoy life and to be free—to relish and explore that freedom to be yourself since "the world was made to be free in." The blind can and shall continue to be free.

## CONCLUSION FOR NOW

We have covered quite a lot of terrain, tracing blindness in literature from ancient Greek epics and tragedies through contemporary novels, and we have examined and analyzed a wide array of blind characters and images of blindness and sight. We have explored imagery relating blindness to ignorance or blind rage and sight to poetic or spiritual vision. The eye is called the window of the soul, and our subtle moods and facial expressions and gestures play a large role as we mature. Learning to flirt, to wink, and how to make confident eye contact are all part of maturing, a part of growing up most of us are unaware of, yet a necessary part of coming into maturity, a part crucial to normal socialization. In this parade of literary texts relating to blindness and the blind, we have covered the gamut of blind in literature and autobiography—the crafty, cold, mean Lazarillo de Tormes and Junko through James Kelman's raunchy, self-blinding protagonist. We have seen good and bad, stereotypical and unique, smart and not-so-smart blind people, and we have noted many of the literary connotations of sight, blindness, and the eye.

## NOTE

1. In the 20th century, in the television series *The Avengers*, the person in charge of covert operations defending Britain's security is called Mother and is a wheelchair-bound man. In one episode as a comic element a second in command is introduced called Father, a blind woman.

# 3

# Original Fiction by the Blind

My darkness has been filled with the light of intelligence, and behold, the outer day-lit world was stumbling and groping in social blindness.

Helen Keller

We have assembled a diverse collection of short stories written by talented blind writers, ranging from a blind girl's adventure while spelunking and her encounter with blind cave fish to the stresses of a blind professional's job interview with a narrow-minded interviewer, from a wedding to an adoption, and a teacher's semiautobiographical account of teaching students how to walk with the blind and the strange anomalies that occur in such classes. Enjoy the read!

## THE ADOPTION

### by Abbie Johnson Taylor

"I'm sorry, but there's nothing more I can do," said the doctor as he turned and left the room.

I looked at my wife, Betty, who lay in her hospital bed, her sightless eyes filling with tears. "Warren," she said, extending her hand in search of mine.

"I'm right here, honey," I said, taking her hand.

As she burst into tears, I took her in my arms and she buried her face in my neck. "Oh, Warren," she sobbed. "I really wanted us to have children. How could this happen to me, to us?"

"I don't know," I said with a sad sigh. "But I don't see any reason why we can't adopt." I straightened and handed her a Kleenex from the box on the nightstand. I brushed back the hair from her eyes as she continued to sob for a few more minutes.

Finally, she blew her nose and said with a note of disdain in her voice, "They wouldn't let a blind woman adopt a baby."

"I don't see why not," I said. "Isn't this Americans with Disabilities Act supposed to protect people like you in situations like this? It helped you a couple of years ago when your boss said she couldn't work with your blindness and reduced your hours."

"I don't know," said Betty with a sigh.

"Look, your lawyer uncle helped you with that battle a couple of years ago," I reminded her. "I'll bet he could help us now if we need him."

"I suppose," said Betty with a yawn.

"Why don't you get some rest," I said. "I'll go get a cup of coffee, and I'll be back soon." I kissed her forehead and left the room.

As I walked down the hall, I thought about the events of the past few months. Betty and I were so excited when we discovered that she was pregnant. I took out a home equity loan and was working with a contractor to build an extra room onto the house for the baby. Some friends of ours offered us a crib and other baby items they no longer needed.

Then last night, Betty started bleeding. I called 911, and she was rushed to the hospital, where she soon miscarried. This morning, they ran some tests to determine the cause of the miscarriage, and we soon learned the sad news. Because of a rare genetic disorder, Betty would never be able to carry a baby to term. The doctor predicted that she would always miscarry during the third month and suggested that we try adoption or some other means of having children.

Now, I stopped in front of the nursery and looked in the window. A baby in a nearby crib caught my attention. Her eyes were blue and her hair was blonde and curly. I felt a twinge of sadness. Would our baby have looked like that? As I watched, the baby began to cry as did others in the room. A nurse hurried to the crib and picked up the baby. She glanced in my direction, and a moment later, the nursery door opened and there she stood, holding the baby who was still whimpering. In bewilderment, I turned toward her.

"Excuse me," she said with an apologetic smile. "I couldn't help but notice you watching this baby."

"Oh, she's not mine," I explained. "You see, my wife had a miscarriage last night and I couldn't help looking at that baby and thinking ours would have probably looked just like that."

"I'm sorry," said the nurse, her face softening with compassion. "But listen, I know this isn't your baby. But I'm the only one back here and there are four other babies who also need attention. And this baby's mother isn't here. Would you mind giving her a bottle?"

I didn't hesitate. "Sure," I said.

As I took the baby from the nurse and followed her into the nursery, I wished it was our baby I was carrying. I sat in a rocking chair in the corner of the room and the nurse handed me a bottle and showed me what to do. She hurried off to tend to the other crying babies and the one in my lap was soon sucking on her bottle. I noticed that this baby's eyes seemed to stare into space the way Betty's eyes did. Could this baby be blind too?

When the room was quiet, the nurse returned and stood watching me. "You do that very well," she said. "I'm so sorry you lost your own baby. You would have been a good father."

"Thanks," I said. "By the way, where is this baby's mother?"

With a sigh, the nurse replied, "She and her husband just left the hospital this morning without the baby."

"You mean they abandoned her?" I asked in astonishment.

"I'm afraid so," said the nurse.

"Why?" I asked in disbelief.

"The baby was born blind," answered the nurse.

"I knew it!" I cried. "My wife's blind too. You mean this baby's parents just left her because she's blind?"

"That's what it looks like," said the nurse. As if she overheard our conversation, the baby in my lap stirred and began whimpering. "She's probably had enough," said the nurse. "Now you need to burp her. Just put her over your shoulder and tap her lightly on the shoulder."

As I did what she instructed, the baby stopped whimpering and the nurse smiled. "Don't worry, sweetheart," I said to the baby. "Daddy's here now."

At this, the nurse raised her eyebrows. I was also taken aback by what I just said. The words seemed to come out of my mouth unbidden. But I realized that fate placed this child who was abandoned by her parents into the arms of a father who just lost a child. Mustering all my courage, I said, "I know this sounds awfully sudden, but how would my wife and I go about adopting this baby?"

The nurse gaped in astonishment. "Let me make a call," she said. As she hurried from the room, I could detect a hint of a smile of approval around the corners of her mouth.

A few minutes later, a dark-haired woman in a business suit came into the room. When she saw me with the baby, her serious face broke into a broad grin. She approached me and extended a hand. "Hi, I'm Vinnessa Cain, and I'm a social worker here," she said in a cheerful tone of voice.

Still holding the baby, who'd fallen asleep, I rose. Cradling her in the crook of my left arm, I extended my right hand. "I'm Warren Foster."

"It's nice to meet you," said the social worker. "I understand you're interested in adopting this baby."

"Yes," I answered. Not knowing how much the nurse told her, I continued, "My wife and I just lost a baby due to a miscarriage, and we just found out that my wife cannot have children."

"I'm so sorry," said the social worker. "But you're in luck today. It just so happens that there's a case worker from the Department of Family Services in my office and we were discussing this particular baby when the nurse up here called me. Why don't you come with me down to my office and talk to her, and she can give you some idea of what would be involved."

I looked down at the sleeping bundle in my arms, hesitant to part company with this baby so soon. "Should I leave her here?" I asked, hoping I would not be forced to abandon this child as she was once before abandoned.

"Let's take her along," answered the social worker. "It's important that DFS workers see how you interact with the child." To reassure me, she said, "I think you're going to make a wonderful father."

I followed the social worker down the hall to the elevator that took us to the ground floor of the hospital. We proceeded through a maze of corridors until we reached an office. All the while, the social worker made pleasant small talk and I tried to sound cheerful when I answered. But a knot of anxiety was developing in my stomach. I knew that first impressions were important and right now, I didn't look very good. I had spent the night in a recliner in Betty's room, and my clothes and hair were rumpled and I was in need of a shave. But the social worker's last words rang in my ear. "I think you're going to make a wonderful father," she'd said. Maybe she was right.

As we walked into the office, a blonde woman in another business suit rose and smiled when she saw me and the baby. "Hi, I'm Annette Barkley with the Department of Family Services," she said.

I cradled the baby and extended my hand and introduced myself. When we'd settled ourselves, she asked, "How did you find out about this baby?"

I explained my wife's blindness and told the story of how Betty and I lost our baby and how we were told that Betty could have no more children. I explained how I walked by the nursery window and noticed this baby. I told how the nurse, flustered because she was the only one on duty and there were several babies needing her attention, asked me to give her a bottle. I told the DFS worker how I fell in love with this baby and how I was moved by the child's plight, which the nurse had explained to me. "I think fate somehow brought us together," I said.

"It certainly sounds like it," the DFS worker mused. "But your wife hasn't seen this baby, has she?"

"No," I answered. "But I know she wants a baby just as much as I do. In fact, she's feeling pretty depressed right now, and so I think this baby will cheer her up."

"You're probably right," replied the DFS worker. "And I'm sure your wife could provide a lot of love and support to a child who is in the same boat as she is. And I can already see that you're going to make a great father. So let's go talk to your wife, shall we?"

As we left the hospital social worker's office and walked down the hall, I felt as if a great weight were lifted from my shoulders. As I glanced down at the baby in my arms, I noticed that she was awake. We took the elevator back up to Betty's floor and walked into her room. Betty was sleeping but, sensing our presence, she woke and her eyes turned toward me. I approached the bed and said, "Honey, I have a surprise for you. Hold out your arms."

Looking bewildered, Betty did as I told her. As the two social workers looked on from the doorway, I placed the baby into her arms. With a look of surprise on her face and tears of joy filling our eyes, Betty's arms encircled the tiny form. The End

Reprinted with permission from Abbie Johnson Taylor.

## THE WEDDING

### *by Abbie Johnson Taylor*

With trepidation, Mark climbed the front porch steps to the old redbrick house and rang the front doorbell. Years ago as a boy, he came to this house almost every day to collect his friend Steve and they walked to school together. Now, he was here on a different mission, and he was wondering if he should have come at all. But for Steve's sake, he had to try.

"Hello, Mrs. Wilson," he said to the woman who opened the door. "I don't know if you remember me, but I'm Mark Bradley. I used to live across the street from you, and Steve and I went to school together."

After a brief pause, Gladys Wilson's face lit up with recognition and she smiled. "Of course! It's been a long time since we've seen you. Come on in."

She led Mark into the living room where Steve's father was reclining in his chair, reading the morning paper. He looked up as Gladys spoke.

"Henry, look who's here. It's Mark Bradley. You remember Mark. He and Steve went to school together, and he lived right across the street."

With a broad grin, Henry rose from his chair, flinging the newspaper aside and offering his hand to Mark. Mark, breathing a little more easily now, shook hands with the older man. "Sit down, Mark," said Henry.

Mark obeyed, taking a chair near Henry's recliner. Henry settled himself back in his chair and picked up the newspaper.

"Henry and I slept in this morning and I was just about to fix us some breakfast," said Gladys. "Are you hungry, Mark?"

"Sure," answered Mark.

"How does bacon, eggs, and toast sound?" asked Gladys.

"Great," replied Mark.

In truth, Mark was not a bit hungry. But he was glad of any excuse to put off stating the real reason for his visit. When he was a boy, he'd shared many meals with the Wilson family. They spent many sleepless nights in Steve's attic bedroom, driving Steve's older sister Sarah to distraction with their noise. The Wilson house became a second home to Mark over the years, and so it felt natural to chat with Henry in the living room and then move into the dining room when the meal was ready.

"I saw your mother in the supermarket not long ago," said Gladys as they ate. "She said that you are now at the School of Mines studying electrical engineering, is that right?"

"Yeah," answered Mark, pushing food around on his plate. "I guess Steve didn't tell you."

Henry put down his fork and sighed. "Steve hasn't spoken to us since I told him I didn't want him marrying that girl that he's marrying today."

"Oh, Henry!" Gladys exclaimed. "I just don't understand why you don't like Kathleen. You haven't even met her. Did Steve tell you, Mark, that he and Kathleen came by one day so we could meet her? When they told us they were coming, Henry insisted we go out somewhere so we wouldn't be home when they got here."

"Gladys, you know very well why I don't approve of Kathleen, and I don't think Mark came over here to listen to us dredge that up again," said Henry, his face growing red with anger.

Ignoring her husband, Gladys said, "As it turned out, when we got home that day, they were still there, waiting for us. They'd just made themselves comfortable in the living room, as if they expected us back any minute, and were watching TV. We'd gone to Perkins for coffee and dessert and I guess we were gone about half an hour."

Mark grinned, remembering the incident as Steve had told it to him. Steve figured his parents were trying to avoid meeting Kathleen on purpose. So thinking Henry and Gladys couldn't stay away from home forever, Steve and Kathleen decided to wait for them.

"Anyway," Gladys continued. "Henry didn't even stop to say hello. He didn't even look at Kathleen. He just marched upstairs to our bedroom and slammed the door. But I stayed downstairs and had a very nice visit with them."

"Gladys, I don't want to talk about this right now," said Henry.

"Kathleen's a very sweet girl," Gladys went on. "And she's amazing! She can't see very well but she can live on her own and hold down a job. And I think it's wonderful that she works in a nursing home and sings to those poor old people there. Sarah says she has a wonderful voice, and isn't it a funny coincidence that Sarah and Kathleen work in the same nursing home? I think Sarah deliberately put Steve and Kathleen together."

"And that's another thing!" exclaimed Henry. "What's Sarah doing wiping old people's bottoms anyway? She should find a husband of her own and settle down."

Ignoring Henry, Mark said, "I think you're right about Sarah putting Steve and Kathleen together. When they met, Steve's band was playing at the Golden Eagle."

"And why is Steve playing that damn rock and roll music?" asked Henry. "When he was growing up, he'd play his drums to my Oscar Peterson record. Now he's playing this stuff that isn't even music."

"Oh, Henry, pipe down," said Gladys in exasperation. Turning to Mark, she said, "Now, what were you saying about Steve playing at the Golden Eagle?"

"Well," continued Mark. "Sarah brought Kathleen to the Golden Eagle to hear Steve play."

"A bar," Henry muttered.

"A nightclub," Mark corrected him with a grin. "Anyway, during a break, Sarah took Kathleen up to the bandstand to meet Steve and they hit it off right away. I was there too that night, and as I recall, during every break after that, Steve went over to the table where Kathleen and Sarah were sitting and visited while Sarah went to the ladies' room. After that night, those two were inseparable. And you know the rest of the story."

"I wonder what Steve saw in that girl," Henry grumbled.

"I think it's their interest in music that brought them together, as well as Sarah's matchmaking, of course," replied Mark. With a wink at Henry, he continued, "And I think you'd be interested to know that Kathleen's been trying to convince Steve to help her form a jazz band that would play some of those old songs at the nursing home."

"I remember that day they were here," said Gladys. "Kathleen said she plays the piano and the guitar and then she also has one of those electronic keyboards."

"Oh, really," said Henry with interest. "But how's she going to take care of Steve? Can she even cook or clean?"

"Kathleen's an excellent cook," answered Mark. "Of course, she has some vision but she does some things by feel. Her stove and oven have raised marks on them to indicate the different settings and temperatures. She's got a talking timer and a talking bread machine. As far as cleaning is concerned, she hires someone to clean for her once a week. Of course, it used to be once every other week until Steve moved in."

"You mean they're actually living together!" exclaimed Henry, his face growing red with anger.

"Well, yeah," said Mark, not knowing what else to say. "Nowadays, finding a wife is like buying a car. You have to test drive it first."

"That's bullshit!" Henry shouted, rising from his chair. His quick movement caused the chair to topple to the floor with a loud thud. "I'm not going to listen to any more of this!" he sputtered as he stamped out of the room. A moment later, his footsteps were heard climbing the stairs to the second floor and a door slammed. Mark noticed that Gladys's face was expressionless.

"I hope my last remark didn't offend you too," he said.

"Not at all," replied Gladys with a note of sadness in her voice. "I suppose that, nowadays, women think the same way about getting husbands," she said with a weak smile.

"Yeah, I guess so," said Mark. Now was the time to state his business. "As Steve's best man, I actually came by today to personally invite you and Mr. Wilson to the wedding."

"Oh," said Gladys, looking startled. "We did get an invitation, and that's another thing Henry doesn't approve of. For some reason, he doesn't like the idea of them getting married at the nursing home. I think it's quite sweet."

"I agree," said Mark. "Kathleen has developed friendships with some of the residents and she says it's like having extra grandparents. So she wants everyone of them who can to attend and the staff as well."

"Sarah told me over the phone that she's going to sing "I'll Take You Home Again, Kathleen" as the bride is coming down the aisle," said Gladys. "Now that's certainly different."

"Well, you see," said Mark, "Kathleen heard Sarah singing that song to one of the residents as she was bathing her and she liked it so much that she asked Sarah to sing it at their wedding, exactly as she sang it in the tub room, without any accompaniment. And instead of saying vows, Steve and Kathleen are going to sing songs to each other, but neither of them knows that the other is doing that. They each think that the other will speak the vows."

"Now that's interesting," said Gladys. She lowered her head and sighed. "I'll talk to Henry. Maybe I can convince him to come. If not, maybe I'll come on my own. I don't know. I'll see." With that, she put her elbows on the table and rested her chin in her hands.

Mark realized that he'd said his piece and it was time to leave. But there was one more thing he could say. "You know, this is one of the most important days in Steve's life. He needs you. Don't you think you should at least attend your own son's wedding?"

Gladys said nothing and did not move. As Mark walked out the front door and slid behind the wheel of his car, he reflected on his visit with Steve's parents. Although he was distressed by Henry's reaction to the situation, he was glad that he'd tried to set things straight between Steve and his parents. Steve did not know that Mark had planned to visit Henry and Gladys, and he never would.

Later that afternoon in the crowded chapel of Pine Ridge Manor, Mark stood with Steve at the altar, waiting for the bride to enter. Mark glanced around the room, hoping that he would spot Henry and Gladys, but he did not see them. With a sinking heart, he looked at Steve to gauge his reaction to the absence of his parents. But by the look on Steve's face, Mark guessed that Steve wasn't thinking about his parents. His eyes were glued to the doorway in anticipation of Kathleen's arrival.

A hush fell over the room and Sarah began to sing. There were the usual bridesmaids and flower girls, and finally, Kathleen came into the room on her father's arm. At least Kathleen's family did not disapprove of her union with Steve. Although they were devout Catholics, they welcomed Steve, despite the fact that he chose not to convert to the religion. They even hired a nondenominational minister to perform the ceremony. Perhaps Mr. and Mrs. O'Brien were glad that someone was willing to marry their disabled daughter. When Kathleen and her father reached the altar, they stopped in front of Steve. Kathleen extended her hand and Steve took it.

As the minister began a short sermon on the meaning of marriage, Mark glanced toward the doorway. He looked again. Sure enough, standing in the doorway were Henry and Gladys Wilson. Mark nudged Steve and pointed. Steve gaped in astonishment. He turned and whispered something to Kathleen, who looked surprised. They were just getting settled as the minister was saying, "If anyone has any reason why this man and this woman should not be joined in holy matrimony, please speak now or forever hold your peace."

Mark held his breath, expecting Henry to say something. But for once, he was silent.

After a pause, the minister announced it was time for Steve and Kathleen to give their vows. Kathleen was to be first. Sarah sat at the piano and played the opening bars of "You Light Up My Life," and Kathleen began to sing. Steve's eyes widened in astonishment. Gladys and a few other women wiped their eyes.

When Kathleen finished her song, Steve whispered to Mark, "Man, I can't do this. I don't sing as well as she does. Tell Sarah not to bother. I'll just say something instead."

But Sarah struck up the opening bars to the song Steve planned to sing, and Steve turned and looked into Kathleen's eyes and began to sing. He hesitated at first but his voice grew stronger. Some of the men wiped their eyes and Kathleen's maid of honor gave her a Kleenex. But Henry remained motionless, with a disgusted scowl on his face. Granted, Steve was a better drummer than a singer but his words were clear. "I hope you don't mind that I put down in words how wonderful life is when you're in the world."

After Steve and Kathleen exchanged rings, the local chapter of Sweet Ade-lines, a women's barbershop group of which Kathleen was a member, filed onto a set of risers. As they sang, "Every day of my life, I'll be in love with you," there wasn't a dry eye in the crowd. Even Henry was wiping his eyes. Mark pulled two handkerchiefs out of his pocket and gave one to Steve. After their song was finished, the minister pronounced Steve and Kathleen man and wife. Kathleen took Steve's arm, and as Sarah played Mendelsohn's "Wedding March," they filed out of the chapel.

The reception was to be held in one of the resident dining rooms. As Mark stood in the receiving line with others in the wedding party, he looked around for Henry and Gladys. Sure enough, there they were. As they drew closer, Mark noticed that both Henry and Gladys were smiling and so was Steve.

"Honey, Mom and Dad are coming," Steve said. "Dad's right in front of you now."

Kathleen extended her hand. "Hello, Mr. Wilson. It's so nice to finally meet you," she said with a note of uncertainty in her voice.

Henry grasped Kathleen's hand and shook it. With a broad grin on his face, he said, "Welcome to the family, Kathleen."

Reprinted with permission from Abbie Johnson Taylor.

\* \* \*

*Marissa, Obstacle Illusions* is Grace D. Napier's semiautobiographical novel about a "present-day educated, employed, independent, resourceful, active blind" woman who is "prominent in society. The novel strips away any mystique about how blind individuals function. The answers are practi-cal, reasonable and straightforward" (*Marissa* back cover). Marissa, a retired professor who still presents her research at academic conferences, would be considered admirably competent even if she were not blind, yet what she does and accomplishes although blind is truly remarkable. She uses every minute of her time effectively and is at the center of a wide circle of gen-erous friends. While the author was seeking to portray a truly phenom-enal woman, one who cares passionately about world affairs and citizens' rights as well as classical music and many other aspects of modern life—addressing all these subjects successfully—it is the little accomplishments that move and fascinate us: for instance, one morning, because it is snow-ing in the town of Spencer, and she's had to cancel all her appointments, Marissa sews in her apartment in a residence for the blind, then swims, and then lifts weights for body strengthening. Napier's purpose seems to be to demystify everything surrounding blindness and to show that this blind woman at any rate is every bit as competent, if not more so, as any other professional woman. Here she describes how her heroine sews:

"Marissa then began to work on some garments that needed mending. Although she could sew by hand, someone with vision had to select the correct shade of thread for her. Spools of thread could be labeled in Braille, but each color had many shades and she could not select the most appropriate shade in relation to the garment and where it would be used. She gathered the items to be repaired: a detached button on this blouse, a loose spot in this skirt's hem, a strap here, the pocket on this apron, and the cuff on this jacket sleeve. When the shade had been selected, Marissa put the garment and spool of thread together until she sat down to sew. Although she herself did not use a sewing machine, she had blind friends who used power machines proficiently. Success in learning hinged on competent teaching. Blind people can thread needles by using either a needle-threader or calyx needles. With the latter, thread is placed across the calyx and then pulled down on both sides until the thread drops inside and the needle is threaded.

"Marissa decided to ask Hope to select the threads. Then she could do the mending this morning and be done with it before lunch."

Later, while mending, Marissa considers how easy mobility is "within Spencer itself because of the cleared sidewalks and plowed streets. By contrast, going on foot outside Spencer was hazardous. Therefore she had no plans to leave the complex today. She liked the sound, however, of going to the warmwater pool after lunch. The exercise would be just what she needed after yesterday's enforced confinement, longer than what Marissa was accustomed to. The hours between one o'clock and three o'clock were reserved for Spencer residents. Afterward, it was available for two hours to townspeople with medical referrals, but she doubted that any of them would travel to the pool that day" (157–58).

At the pool, she meets a friend and ties her Labrador service dog nearby so he can watch her enjoying an invigorating swim in the nearly empty pool. Afterward, she lifts dumbbells in her apartment and speaks on the phone with a gentleman named Dan who has just sent her flowers and wants to send her an airline ticket so she can come visit him.

A creative, intelligent professor, she teaches general-studies students how to work with the blind, even though the students are not intending to make working with the blind their careers. Earlier in the novel, she had described to Dan what and how she teaches them:

"Seated in the living room again, Marissa said, 'I must clarify to you, Dan, that the blind person doesn't always have to be on your right side. [Previously she had trained Dan to walk with a blind person by teaching him how to give her essential directions clearly.] Either side works equally well, except when the blind person's guide is an amputee! Let me digress to relate an experience that occurred in one of my classes.

"'I was teaching a survey course primarily for students who were not planning to work in the field of blindness. In this course, we covered many topics to familiarize students with the field of visual impairment. This day we were discussing orientation and mobility—called O&M for short. When talking about the human guide, I asked for a volunteer. A male student came forward and stood to my left, asking, "Does it matter which side of you I stand on?" My reply was that either side works equally well. He stayed on my left. When I reached for his right arm, [though,] I did not find it. He was a military amputee, which fact I had not known until that moment. He was a good sport to volunteer to place himself in that situation. I don't know whether he had assumed that I knew, because I knew his name (and voice) and had chatted with him before that morning, or whether he had assumed that I did not know but he wanted to see how I would deal with the circumstances.'

"'How did you deal with the surprise?'

"'I said that I would go behind him to his other side and use his left arm. Now let us return to the situation when you are walking with a person who has a dog guide on his/her left side. Then that person needs to be on your left.'

"'Why would the blind person be holding my arm when she has a dog?'

"'That's a valid question, Dan. Suppose you and I are going to meet for dinner some evening, but I meet you, say, at the bus stop where I get off after having attended a meeting. Maybe you use the same bus stop but different bus, getting off after leaving your worksite. Then we walk to the restaurant. I have my dog with me. If I continue to use her while you and I are talking en route to the restaurant, I can confuse her. [For instance] When I agree with what you are saying, I say, "Right!" The dog thinks I'm giving her a command. Or I tell you about someone who left his wife and children, and the dog hears "left" and thinks it's a command.'

"'Now I understand why. Thanks for the explanation. I hope I don't forget all this by the next time we are together.' . . .

"'You might have occasion to use these skills to help a person other than me,' Marissa pointed out. 'Someone may need help to cross the street. You can say, "May I help you?" Let him tell you what kind of help he needs, if any. Don't assume you know. If you are to take him somewhere, say, "Take my arm"'" (Napier 77–78).

This lucid novel is filled with great advice on how to help, walk with, and work with the blind and their dog guides. It is almost a blind manual of etiquette and is a must-read for anyone learning to go out in public with a blind person or for someone newly blind who may need to know what he or she may expect to be able to do. According to Napier, the blind can easily travel alone safely and do virtually anything they want to. After all, her subtitle is *Obstacle Illusions*, implying that any obstacles are illusions.

Reprinted with permission from Grace D. Napier.

* * *

Short story writer Chris Kuell writes more traditional short stories and integrates much humor into every story.

## JUST CALL ME AL

### *by Chris Kuell*

The jingle of the bell at the door caught me off guard. I was squatting in a very unladylike position, tightening a nut on the new trap in the double sink. Twenty past eleven was early, even for the biker crowd. I heard the tap, tap, tap of a cane and stood up to see Mike Edison, a blind frequenter of my bar, The Chicken Bone Café. He made his way to the corner stool, collapsed his cane and tucked it under his leg.

"Hey, Mike. Haven't seen you much this summer. What've you been up to?"

"Oh, you know, the usual," he said. "Training for the Olympics—I'm pole vaulting this year. I'm also taking a welding class at the Voc."

"Smart aleck," I said, and poured him a pint.

"Actually, I've been making good progress on my novel. I'm on Chapter 17, a little over 200 pages."

"Hey, that's great," I said. "Congratulations." I placed the beer on a coaster in front of him. He reached out at the sound and found the glass.

"So, why are you in here before eleven-thirty, instead of home, writing a steamy sex scene?"

"Well, I came down here for some inspiration from my favorite bartender."

"Nice try," I said. "You and the wife arguing?" Mike lived down the street, so he came to the Chicken Bone sometimes to cool down and gain perspective.

"No, that's not it," he said. He took a long pull on his beer. "Lisa and I are O.K." Mike took another drink, and then looked me right in the chest. Now, I know he can't see, and he doesn't know that is where his gaze is focused. But at times, I have to wonder.

"You ever notice how I have a knack for irritating people?"

"That's not true, Mike," I said. "You seem to get along with everybody—especially when you're buying."

I turned on the faucet and checked the new pipe for leaks, but everything was dry.

"There was that one night, though, when I thought I was going to have to take the baseball bat to you and Steve. You'd had too much to drink and were quite vocal in your opinion about jobs, or something like that."

"I wasn't drunk," he broke in. "I was just angry. That guy was blabbering about his tax dollars going to support disabled people, taking away their incentive to work. His skull is too thick to understand that blind people want to work. They are just as capable, but nobody will give them the opportunity."

His face reddened and he stopped talking. After another sip of beer, he said, "Well, I irked a lot of people in the Internet writers' group I belong to by posting an angry response to a lady who asked why the state should have to buy accessible voting machines, when people were always there to assist anyone who needs help." Mike sighed, then continued. "I am tired of working so hard to convince people that, most of the time, I can do things myself. By keeping us dependent, the sighted world continues the myth that we are incapable."

"What didn't they like?"

He drained his beer, and I poured him another. Nobody else had come in yet, so I didn't mind talking.

"Some people said it was ridiculous. America didn't have to bow to pressure from special interest groups. As long as help was provided, we have nothing to complain about." Mike paused for a moment. "I admit I overreacted, but I thought my argument was logical. I hoped maybe, just maybe, my words would make people think seriously about how frustrating it is to be perpetually treated like a child. To have the simplest things held just outside your grasp."

"Doesn't sound bad to me." I warmed up the small grill where I made burgers and sandwiches for the lunch crowd.

"I didn't think it was. After I posted it, I thought of a dozen other points I should have included. You can guess how it went. The choir cheered, and the rest wished the blind guy would go away."

"I try never to discuss politics with people unless I know where they stand," I said. "It's just asking for trouble. You want a burger?"

"Sure," he said. "You're wrong, though. The issues aren't just political; there are societal misconceptions that must be changed. And, I get so weary of the lip service. Somebody's got to say something." He sipped and scratched the nubs of beard on his face.

"Un-hunh," I said, flipping the burger.

Mike sat quietly, the sizzling of hamburger the only sound in the bar.

"You know what I was thinking about this morning when I was eating my cereal?"

"What?"

"I remind myself of Al Sharpton, which is not a compliment." He shook his head and rubbed one finger along the edge of his glass. "Now, I'm no fan of Mr. Sharpton. He is a bigot who takes up causes primarily to get his face on TV. But, even though nobody of power takes him seriously, they have to listen, to appease him somehow, because he does have followers. In his loudmouthed, opportunistic, wacko kind of way, he brings attention to African American issues—and people notice."

The door jingled with the arrival of fresh patrons. I set the burger down in front of Mike.

"Ketchup at ten o'clock," I said, putting down a bottle.

"Reagan's favorite vegetable," he said. He felt for the top of the hamburger bun and splashed a glob left of center.

"It makes everybody's buns taste better."

I laughed. "Do you ever stop thinking about sex, Mike?"

"Sure. I only think about sex 45 out of every 60 seconds. Gotta leave some time for politics, religion, and general daydreaming."

"Personally," I said, pouring a beer for another customer, "I think you should carve out more time for your book, and spend less time gabbing with your friends on e-mail. Biggest time waster ever invented."

"You're right," he said. "But, writing is a lonely business. I don't go to an office where I can interact with other people around the coffee machine."

He finished his burger and wiped his hands and mouth with a napkin.

"Another beer, Mike?" I asked.

"No," he said, reaching in his pocket and handing me a 20, folded neatly into a triangle. "You've convinced me. I'm going back to my novel, where I can at least pretend ignorance is fixable."

"After you finish, you can have a book signing here," I said.

"That ought to bring in two or three new customers," he said.

I handed him his change. He said, "Keep the ones and just give me the five."

"Mike, that's about a 40 percent tip," I said.

"Support your local bartender," he announced to the two other patrons, and then got up to leave.

I held the door and he pinched me as he walked by. I gave him a quick jab to the shoulder, but he shrugged it off and laughed.

Two college-age girls watched Mike tap his way down the street. They came into the bar, bubbling with excitement.

"Hey, was that guy the blind writer?" one of the girls asked.

"Yes," I said. "But he thinks he's Al Sharpton."

Reprinted with permission from Chris Kuell.

Here's another, more sardonic story by Chris Kuell.

## HOOK IN HER HEAD (THE INTERVIEW)

### *by Chris Kuell*

The pleasant receptionist tapped lightly three times on the office door, opened it a few inches, and said, "Excuse me, Mrs. Carlisle. Your nine o'clock interview, Robin Simms, is here."

Robin detected no response from within the office, but the receptionist told her to go on in.

"Thank you," Robin replied, and then said in a lower voice, "Forward." A few steps inside the small room, Robin stopped next to a large desk. Taking a deep breath, she smiled and said, "Hello, I'm Robin Simms."

No sound indicated the presence of Mrs. Carlisle. Robin subconsciously checked the top buttons on her blouse. All O.K. Then she ran her fingers through her hair, which seemed perfectly in place.

"Hello?" she tried again.

A pensive, two-pack-a-day voice a few feet in front of her said, "I'm Nancy Carlisle."

Robin stepped forward, hitting her thigh lightly on the wooden desk. She put out her hand, and Nancy Carlisle accepted it weakly, as if she were touching a dead fish. An awkward few seconds followed.

Robin said, "Pleasure to meet you." In a lower voice, she said, "Sid, chair." Her dog walked her two feet to the left and stopped. Robin's probing fingertips encountered the rough cloth of an office chair. She sat while commanding Sid to lie down, and pressed her skirt neatly across her lap.

Another painful pause ensued. The tick, tick, tick of a clock was clearly audible.

"Are you blind?" asked Mrs. Carlisle. It seemed to Robin that the woman's voice was on the verge of incredulity.

"Yes, I am," Robin answered matter-of-factly.

"You didn't say in your cover letter or resume that you were blind." Now the tone was moving toward aggressive. Less than 60 seconds, Robin thought, a new world record.

"I didn't mention I was five foot four or a Methodist, either. With only one page, I prefer to just list my skills and qualifications." The words spilled out before Robin could stop them. She clamped her teeth shut to extinguish any more sarcastic comments.

"Well, don't you think it would be appropriate?" Mrs. Carlisle spat back at her. "Not only have you caught me unprepared, I just, ahh, we, ahh, don't have any jobs here that would be appropriate for a, ah, visually handicapped person."

The old human resources training was kicking in, ever careful to be politically correct. Robin unclenched her jaw and said, "I'm blind. Let's just say it like it is. I apologize for catching you off guard, it wasn't my intent to put you off balance. If you have my resume, you can see that I have a perfect background for the financial analyst position you advertised in the paper. My blindness is not an issue; my skills and work ethic are."

She took a breath, hoping that had come out all right.

"Is that a guide dog?"

Oh boy, here we go with the amazing dog questions, Robin thought. Let's change the topic from my skills to the puppy.

"Yes, this is Sid. He helps me get around."

"Where did you get him—one of them guide dog schools?"

At least the woman was curious. Maybe things would lighten up and then they could proceed.

"Yes, I got him at a school in New York," Robin replied.

"How much did he cost?"

Well, she scores two points for directness, Robin thought.

"I didn't have to pay for him. The school has endowments and grants to pay for the dogs and training. From what I understand, they cost about twenty thousand dollars."

"Taxpayers' money?" Mrs. Carlisle snorted, followed by a short rumbling cough.

Robin didn't take the bait, saying instead, "I don't know," and leaving it at that.

Another awkward pause filled the room with tension. Robin felt a droplet of perspiration rolling down her back. It was hot in this suit. This wasn't going well, and a part of her just wanted to run away. Yet, she really needed this job, hell, any job at this point.

This one was perfect though. The position was for an assistant financial analyst, for which Robin was actually overqualified. She had a bachelor's degree in business, with a minor in accounting. Their office was only a block from the bus line, so at least transportation would be manageable. She crossed her fingers, which were folded in her lap, and silently prayed the interview would improve.

A rustling of papers came from Mrs. Carlisle's desk. More silence, tick, tick, tick.

"Who did your resume for you?"

Irritation, like tinder as it first begins to ignite, began to burn inside Robin.

"I did it myself," Robin said.

"How? Shouldn't it be in Braille or something?"

Robin gave a short chuckle, her turn to be amazed. "I have a computer equipped with speech software at home. It allows me to do word processing, surf the Internet, use spreadsheet programs—most anything a sighted person could do."

More shuffling of papers. Sid got up, panting and wagging into Robin's leg, indicating that he had to go. Oh, not now, Robin thought. Softly but firmly she commanded, "Sid, down." The obedient lab complied.

"I'm impressed to see that you graduated college Ms. Simms, and I'm all in favor of the disadvantaged matriculating into society. I'm sure you are an intelligent woman. But realistically, this is a small firm, and each of our employees is expected to contribute a 110 percent. We don't have the time or the manpower to have people helping you to do whatever amount of work you might be able to accomplish."

With those words, despair settled on the young blind woman. That was it; she had no hope. She was being dismissed, without an ounce of consideration. This whole trip was going to be a waste of time.

"Listen, Mrs. Carlisle. I graduated from college with a 3.6 GPA. All regular classes, I didn't get any breaks. I've interned in the finance department at Shultz & Sons for six months, and they will give me a glowing recommendation. I have great computer skills; I won't need anyone to help me. If I get this job, I can get adaptive computer software and some training in where things are and how things are done. It won't take much, I can learn everything in no time." Robin felt like her voice was a little more pleading toward the end than she would have wished.

"Who's going to take you to the bathroom?" Mrs. Carlisle asked.

Robin sat, completely dumbfounded. Mrs. Carlisle couldn't have shocked her any more if she said she was the love child of Elvis. Was this for real? Do people like this really exist in the world? Unfortunately, Robin knew they did, and worse.

"I've been going to the bathroom without any help since I was three."

"Who helps you?"

Robin wished she could see the agitation that she could sense in Mrs. Carlisle's face.

Mrs. Carlisle, however, was a trained professional and wasn't about to let this blind woman get the better of her. She moved on.

"We have our own computers here, with special software. What makes you think your computer will work with it?" Her tone was as flat and cold as a parking lot in winter.

"I would use your computers, equipped with speech software either provided by the state, your company, or me. The software might have to be customized to work with your programs, but if you are using either Axapta or Navision, I already have the scripts and could be working in a few hours."

These were the programs Robin used at Shultz. Amy Lopez, the woman who installed JAWS and updated the appropriate scripts on her computer for her internship, could also do it here.

Without losing a beat, the interviewer came in with her next question. "How are you going to read mail and paperwork?"

Robin couldn't tell for sure, but she imagined Mrs. Carlisle was sneering. Sid was up again, rubbing against her and wiggling his backside. Robin patted him on the head, saying, "Sit for a little while longer, boy, good boy." Then she focused her attention on the hopeless Mrs. Carlisle.

"That depends. Of course, e-mail is a great medium for a blind person, and as an added benefit it saves paper."

A noticeable exhalation came from Mrs. Carlisle, but Robin continued.

"Printed text can usually be scanned, and then I can use the computer to read it. I have a PDA with speech for my personal notes, and I can use Braille for a variety of other note-taking tasks."

"I suppose that is all well and good," Mrs. Carlisle interrupted, "but what about a handwritten memo? What if I write you a note to redo the Smith calculations for 1994? How could you read it?"

This witch was just being confrontational, Robin thought.

"You wouldn't have to leave me a note. You could send me an e-mail, or better yet, just leave me a phone mail. It's not a problem that is insurmountable."

Mrs. Carlisle made some sort of exasperated sound, which was followed by three light knocks on the closed office door. It opened, and a cheery voice said, "Mrs. Carlisle, Mr. Pastor needs to see you in the managers' meeting. He said it was important." Without excusing herself or even acknowledging the existence of the person in her office, Mrs. Carlisle got up from her desk and scurried out the door.

Robin was overcome with a feeling of depression and insignificance. This was painful and there was really no point in continuing with the charade. Robin got out of her chair, and on an impulse reached out and felt the cool, smooth surface of Nancy Carlisle's desk. She tapped it, a heavy, solid sound. Feeling like a kid with her hand in the cookie jar, Robin walked around the desk and sat in the comfy leather high-backed chair. She leaned forward and ran her fingertips over the blotter, keyboard, Rolodex, and flat screen monitor. How could an idiot like Nancy Carlisle ever get such a magnificent desk? What could she possibly do any better than Robin could do, except see? And what gave her the right to treat Robin with such disrespect, like she was trash on the sidewalk?

Slowly, a devious smile crept across Robin's face. She called out, "Sid, come."

A minute later, Robin bid the friendly receptionist a good day as she left the front of the building. What she had hoped would be her first real job wasn't going to be happening here. Oh, well, she thought.

Maybe next time.

Reprinted with permission from Chris Kuell.

\* \* \*

It is intriguing to find John Reiff speaking in a feminine persona in the short story "Cave Fish," where the fish may symbolize the blind female spelunker and narrator herself. We particularly liked his use of unusual words like "echoic" and his description of this arduous and adventurous activity.

## CAVE FISH

### by John Reiff

The cave floor feels smooth beneath my gloved hands and hard under my knees. I can touch either side of the horizontal shaft by extending my arms about a foot out from the shoulders. If I lift my helmeted head 18 inches, I'll bang the ceiling. It's pretty tight. No one talks. The labored, asynchronous breathing of five pairs of lungs mingles with the scraping of five pairs of shin pads on rock. For me, there is total darkness as opposed to the usual sliver of vision available in my right eye. I can sometimes take advantage of that little bit of sight to help me get around outside during the day or in a well-lit room. Not here. The helmet lamp is of no value. I feel my way, follow the sounds made by the others, and heed their occasional prompts and warnings. They bring plenty of light and follow it almost like a religion.

I plunked down $45 on a whim. *Introductory Spelunking.* Three hours in a cave. What was I thinking? I'm 28. Been blind two years. Damn diabetes. Damp brown hair protrudes from my helmet and sticks to my left cheek and throat. Bra straps dig into my bony shoulders with each back and forth arm movement. Should've worn the sports bra. The folding cane swings freely from my belt. Don't think I'm going to need it down here.

"Let's rest a minute" says Rita, our guide. "How's everybody doin'?"

"Doin' great," responds the guy in line just ahead of me. His name is Dan. His speech lacks any recognizable accent.

"Next section goes downhill at a pretty steep angle," she continues. "We'll take it feet first on our butts."

"I got no pad on my butt" cracks Bozo behind me.

"You got plenty of padding on your butt," says his girlfriend, Mary, behind him. I like her.

"How high's the ceiling?" I ask.

"Short arm's length. Use it to push yourself along or break yourself. Is everyone ready?"

"Yeah," we say in unison.

"Let's go."

Ten minutes later the floor levels out and we enter a much larger space, judging by the echoic quality of Rita's voice.

"This is Stella's Grotto. Let's move to the right along the edge of the pool. Notice the columns running from floor to ceiling. The pool contains a small population of eyeless, albino cavefish. Eyes offer no advantage down here since there's no light to see by. The fish use smell, tactile sensory organs to detect movement, and possibly sonar to locate food that drifts in on the underground stream that feeds the pool."

I sense an awkward curtain of silence descending and feel obliged to step up and cast it off.

"That's amazing. I'd like to have sonar ability. I wouldn't have to remember where I left my cane. .... Can I, uh, feel the water?"

"No. Sorry." says Rita. "Oil from your hands would change the chemistry. Wouldn't be good for the fish. Let's move on."

Twenty more minutes of crawling. My knees and the palms of my hands protest each time they touch the floor. Bozo obviously shares my pain.

"Don't we ever get to stand up in here?" he asks.

I sense a smile framing Rita's reply.

"We saved the best for last. There's a few interesting challenges ahead. We'll descend a short, vertical shaft, cross a five-foot, planked crevice, and then a somewhat shorter crevice. After that we're home free. We'll pretty much walk the rest of the way."

"Hallelujah," Bozo responds with obvious relief.

The vertical shaft turns out to be a hole in the floor.

"You gotta be kiddin' me," I comment as I try to measure the diameter of the hole with my hands and compare it with the breadth of my shoulders. We're gonna fit in there?"

"One at a time," says Rita. "Who's first?"

"I'll do it," I blurt brashly.

"When you get to the bottom, move ahead into the horizontal shaft to make room for the rest of us."

I drop my legs into the hole and slowly lower myself to the armpits. I can't feel the bottom. A wave of anxiety erupts within my chest cavity. I'm breathing rapidly.

"Does it get any narrower than this?" I ask, afraid that I sound as nervous as I feel.

"No, pretty much the same all the way to the bottom."

"How far?"

"You'll be there before you know it."

I go. It's O.K. as long as I'm moving. When I hesitate, fear simmers, threatens to boil over, expand, and wedge me in forever. I bottom out after what seems like five or six feet and enter the horizontal shaft, which opens wide enough to easily accommodate three people side by side though still no more than four feet high. The others join me slowly, one at a time.

Rita takes the lead again. We arrive at the first crevice 15 minutes later. She describes the plank bridge and how best to traverse it. Dan goes first on his hands and knees and is across in less than 10 seconds. My turn. I grip the edges, my hands about 18 inches apart, a little less than the width of my shoulders.

"How far is the drop?" I ask.

"About eight feet," Rita replies.

"Great."

I edge out with my knees touching. Easy enough. The plank is thick and firm. It instills confidence. I slide my right hand six inches forward followed by left knee, left hand, right knee. Repeat five times. I'm across. Not bad.

"Last crevice," Rita announces. "Who wants to go first?"

Bozo crawls up. His real name is Marsh, he told us when we all introduced ourselves at the beginning of the day.

"Looks easy," he says. "Where's the plank?"

"No plank, unless you want to go back and get the one we just used. We call this the plankless crevice."

I think she's smiling again.

"I don't get it," Bozo says.

"I'll demonstrate."

The next thing you know, she's across. I have no idea what she did and say so.

"Sorry." She returns to our side. "You need to bring your knees right to the edge and kneel up straight. Bend a little at the waist, reach out slowly with both hands, and fall forward until you connect with the other side. Then it's just a matter of walking forward on your hands a ways and swinging your legs across. You wanna try?"

"O.K." I get into position, bend at the waist, reach out, and freeze.

"Not gonna work!" I say. "Can't do it that way. But I have an idea." I remove my folding cane from my belt and put it together. I find the far edge of the crevice with the tip, fix it there, and slide my one hand down the cane to the tip and solid rock beneath. The other hand acts in concert. I scamper across. The small group behind me cheers. "No way," I say, smiling. "No way in hell I was gonna do that without knowing where my hands were coming down. Mmmm. Mmmm. Don't wanna miss."

"Nice job," says Rita.

"Thanks."

Long day. Good day. Back at the apartment, I treat myself to a hot bath to chase away the damp chill I picked up along with all the dirt. Water laps my neck as I settle into the most comfortable position possible. I think about the eyeless fish that live in a world where vision is impractical in the absence of light and the people who brought light into that dark place in order to find their way.

I consider my cane and how its use enabled me to find the far side of the crevice and get across. I reach up and turn on the hot water to reheat my bath. I'm gonna stay in the tub a bit longer than usual today.

John Reiff
3020 Roosevelt Street
Wall Township, New Jersey 07719
732-681-1346

# 4

❖

# The Blind Writing about Blindness

To be blind is not miserable; not to be able to bear blindness, that is miserable.

John Milton

I did it to myself. It wasn't society . . . it wasn't a pusher, it wasn't being blind or being black or being poor. It was all my doing.

Ray Charles

The following anonymously submitted prose piece that came to us as a result of a posting on the *Braille Forum* expresses much about the experience of blindness and becoming blind.

## AN INTROSPECTION ON BLINDNESS

It is now time to leave behind our negative thinking about blindness and to focus on some of the positive aspects of having a visual impairment. Often when one cannot see, it forces one to attain an introspective quality. If you can no longer look at the visual world, why not look inside instead? Learn to use the other senses and explore the wonder of touch, smell, taste, and hearing. Those senses will expand and enhance every moment.

To concentrate on hearing can be a beautiful experience. Music sounds more beautiful. Often differences in instruments and musical notes are more prevalent. We tune in to other conversations and learn to tell how a person is feeling by the inflection in his or her voice and in the cadence of words. The response to "How are you?" takes on a different meaning when one is really listening to the tone of "Fine." This new understanding can create more compassion, empathy, and understanding.

When we hear, we learn to separate sounds—the sounds of children playing, birds singing, people conversing, cars gliding along, the wind rustling, people walking and talking: sounds come in all at once, not separate, but together, all at the same time. Much of this is never noticed when we are totally in the visual world. Words have more meaning and sounds have more significance now that I am blind.

Touch becomes more important. A hand on your arm means as much or more than a smile did. A guiding shoulder signifies reassurance and comfort. Hands joined in prayer bring us closer to God. A pat on the back means everything is going well.

Our senses of taste and smell become more acute, and we appreciate food more, tasting it more fully. We can recognize our environment more easily. A pharmacy smells different from a bookstore, for example. We probably didn't notice those differences in the past.

And what about being with ourselves? Yes, we have more time for that, and look at what wonder we can find and what emotions we can release. We can experience our emotions more strongly and deeply rather than just brushing them aside. We can enjoy the spoken word of a book more intimately than just reading it. We can learn compassion both for ourselves and for others. We can fully engage in conversations without being outwardly visually distracted. We can pay attention to a lecture without watching everyone else. We can appreciate the sounds of nature and feel natural energy more fully. We can be closer to the universe and the Creator and depend on Him more than on ourselves.

Patti Cataruzolo of Watertown, Massachusetts, contributed "Light," a testament to the great sensory powers and deeper humanity of the blind, for our book. This original, as yet unpublished, poem seems to sum up the sentiments of many of the blind.

Light

Sighted people do not know
the way the sightless come and go,
They seldom seem to understand
what light can be in this dark land...
Where ears can hear and noses smell
much more than sight could ever tell,
Where touch and taste give answers true

to questions sight may "think" it knew;
Better senses, some believe,
are those four left…can't conceive
That better *use* of sense remaining
makes the world a place for gaining
Knowledge, understanding, strength…
I surely could go on at length,
But best I stop and leave with you
The thought I hope I've gotten through…
That though they "see" less with the eye,
They "see" much more than you and I.

Many blind people are convinced that their other senses are stronger than normally sighted people's by way of compensation. And Patti Cataruzolo expresses that successfully and succinctly here.

Reprinted with permission from Patti Cataruzolo.

Next, Nancy Scott of Easton, Pennsylvania, writes a compelling account of the value of her writing for herself and others:

## WHY DO I WRITE?

### *by Nancy Scott*

People often ask me why I've chosen writing as a career, especially since writing and possible publication requires so much working with print. After 335 published pieces, here I am to think about this on paper. These thoughts are in no particular order.

I write to influence and motivate myself and other people. I want to change people's consciousness by raising the particular to the universal. If I find encouragement or fascination, others might benefit from my written observations. I can force awareness and reflection. I can make people laugh or cry. I can explore truths. And I want my truths to stay in my readers' bodies and minds.

I write to figure things out. Writing can focus thoughts in a way that thinking may not. Writing is a form of meditation. Are you more honest when you write? Have you ever written something that you didn't know you knew until you wrote it down?

I write to preserve emotional states and actual memories. Sometimes, I want historical accuracy.

Sometimes, I create a new history rather than keep the old one. Your purpose will tell you how much actual fact is necessary. For instance, I have a poem about my mother's attitude toward her life and death. Her headstone epitaph in the poem is the one I wanted engraved rather than the one she actually has. This will annoy my brother, who doesn't like such poetic license. But the poem's epitaph serves my funnier truth about my mother.

I write to be known, and through art, I can be heard safely. As long as I write, I will never be powerless.

I write to level the playing field. Writing is something I can do. It allows me not to be ignored or invisible as a person who is blind. Writing legitimizes me and what I say. It might even make me famous.

Writing as a blind person forces me to focus on what's important. How many able-bodied writers do you know who put off finishing and mailing that manuscript? They think their time and resources are limitless.

Writing is my identity. People know me as a writer. Grocery checkout clerks say they've read my latest newspaper column. People send me notes after local articles are published. Strangers recognize my name at poetry readings and disability events. I never tire of knowing that people read my work. And, sometimes, I get paid.

Writing is the best work I've ever done. Knowing you're doing your best at something is important. My absolute passion and energy must be on that page. Tomorrow, we can revise it or file it away or send our voice into the world. Next year, we might wish we'd done more editing before it got published. But we must be committed to shaping and telling the best truth we can at the time.

I read somewhere that nothing we write is wasted. It's practice. Some pieces will never be finished. Some things will practically write themselves. Some manuscripts will sit in a file for years and then get pulled out one day and the gold that they are will be obvious.

I want to be the author you keep on your shelf and read at two in the morning. I want to be the book you reread when you need hope. We've all kept books like that. Surely, with practice, we can write them.

Writing is my spiritual path. Sometimes, the distraction of writing absorbs me. Sometimes, the discipline of writing attracts me. More often, the magic of writing amazes me. Writing is what I'm supposed to do. Writing has brought me people when I needed them. It has given me experiences that I was compelled to share on paper.

I think I also read somewhere that, for writers, the rest of your life happens so you can write about it. I now always think of audience. Writing pulls me into and out of my own life.

I write for goals and deadlines and for other people. Editors ask me for articles and I almost can't resist. Writing magazines give me market lists full of ideas. I want 15 bylines this year. Friends expect birthday cards written by me. Some of these cards have gone on to be published pieces. People who help and believe in me make me believe in myself and work harder. My readers bug me if too much time passes and they haven't seen me in print.

Writing is paying attention on paper. This attention ties me to the solid world. It makes me want to stay and participate in that world.

Writing allows a special connection between author and reader. My work has also provided connections between disabled and nondisabled people. There are things I could never say talking to people that I can say on paper. And there are things I need to say that I haven't found the right written words for yet.

Sometimes, I'm afraid I'm not on the right track at all. But I give my best and trust the Universe and keep writing. You can do that, too. And it might lead to your purpose and passion.

Reprinted with permission from Nancy Scott.

Our next writer, Janet Perez Eckles, lives in Orlando, Florida, with "the love of her life, her husband Gene. In addition to a serving as a Sunday school teacher, Jan is an inspirational speaker, writer, and author of *Trials of Today, Treasures for Tomorrow: Overcoming Adversities in Life.*"

## REFLECTION IN THE MIRROR

### *by Janet Eckles*

Out of habit, I felt for the light switch in our bathroom. I flipped it on, but... the darkness remained. My body shook with terror. Holding on to the cold and slick countertop, I looked toward the mirror and saw a dreary gray of nothing. In desperation, I felt the urge to scratch through the glass into the darkness to find even a slight glimpse of my reflection.... Instead, I found the ugliness of my black world.

My blindness entered into my life with a vicious force, ripping apart the dreams my husband, Gene, and I had. Our focus was on raising our three small sons and living happily ever after.

But the unavoidable effects of a retinal disease with no possible cure turned our joy to bitterness and fear.

Motivated by desperation, I began a relentless search for a cure. My visits to fortunetellers, psychics, and New Age healers caused my bank account to diminish and my frustration to increase.

My despair touched those around me. A friend called. "How are you doing?" she asked, concerned about what she knew I was going through.

"Just fine," I lied. The truth was, I was frustrated, hopeless, desperate, and defeated. I was everything but fine.

She continued, "Well, I didn't know how you felt but our church is having a healing service, which I think you might like."

There was my answer—the miracle I longed for! I would be certain to be one of those lucky people and be healed. I welcomed this invitation as a much-needed intermission for the wrestling match of my emotions. But instead, this experience hurled me into the mat of discouragement and deeper anguish. The services proved useless. No healing. No miracle.

"Why, God?" I asked over and over again.

While attending the services, my eyes poured tears and my mind, irrational thoughts. I thought, chances are everyone present was burdened with some degree of personal problems, but none could be as bad as mine. I resented all those who attended. Unlike me, all were sighted and were able to jump into their cars and carry on with their lives. They all could see and thus were more than capable to resolve whatever their issues were. They could see! But me, what chance did I have to move forward?

My heart became much like the metal folding chair I sat on, cold, hard, and lifeless. But in a subtle and unexpected way, the first breath of life entered my soul. It stopped the pounding of my heart. And with a mixture of power and gentleness, this verse forced me to look up: "Seek first the Kingdom of God and His righteousness, and all these things shall be added unto you" (Matthew 6:33 NIV).

A quick sigh slipped from my lips, and my sobbing stopped. What I heard entered my heart, like a floodlight revealing every detail of the source of my pain; I had been consumed with the desperate desire to see again. This was my priority number one; nothing else mattered. But God instructed otherwise, to seek Him first.

Seek Him first? But how!?

The answer came in one word: decision. I had a choice: to continue to sink into my sorrow or look up, open my heart, and see what God would do. I chose the latter; I accepted Jesus as my Savior, my Lord, and my all. The promise I had just heard in this verse warmed my heart like a soft blanket, removing the cold shiver of desperation.

The miracle I hoped for finally became mine. I released with relief, surrendered, and let go the bitterness, pain, and anguish. I saw the evidence of this renewed outlook back home with my little ones. The proof of a transformed heart was reflected in a renewed attitude toward my family, my husband, and life itself.

I recalled the time I anguished at being unable to see my reflection in the mirror. But now, with new eyes, I perceived a new image—a portrait painted with the splendor of God's love, the vibrant colors of His sustaining power, and framed with the golden reassurance of His promises.

I have no sight, but through Christ, I have insight to impart inspiration and hope.

Story courtesy of Janet Perez Eckles, author and inspirational speaker, www.janetperezeckles.com.

Author of *Trials of Today, Treasures for Tomorrow*—a true story of triumph, with practical steps to conquer adversity, heartache, and fear. Now available in audio: http://www.janetperezeckles.com/store.html.

Booktrailer: http://www.tangle.com/view_video?viewkey=6d4decc2f50b21ca652c. Facebook: http://www.facebook.com/people/Janet-Perez-Eckles/664713948. Twitter: http://twitter.com/janeteckles.

Our next writer, DeAnna Quietwater Noriega of Colorado Springs, Colorado, has submitted this poignant piece on her mother and how her mother raised her.

## WIND BENEATH MY WINGS

### *by DeAnna Quietwater Noriega*

My mother was only 17 when I was born. I was the first of her five children. Six months after my birth, I was diagnosed as suffering from congenital glaucoma. The prognosis was not good. My mother was told that I would probably be totally blind by age 10.

Back then, many of the surgical techniques that are used successfully today did not exist. The primary treatment then was a course of drugs administered in eyedrops to control the pressure inside the eye. With each uncontrolled rise in pressure, irreversible damage was done as the lens within the eye was forced back against the delicate retina, destroying rods and cones necessary for vision. Unlike the adult-onset glaucoma, the congenital form is quite painful.

Three operations to stabilize my condition were attempted between the ages of five and eight. The last of these left me without light perception, totally blind.

By that time, I had two normally sighted brothers, respectively two and four years younger than me. My mother had no experience to guide her in rearing a visually impaired child. She had never known a blind person, nor were there any experts to turn to for advice. I was a lively child, curious about everything and independent in temperament. Mom decided that since she knew so little, the best plan was to stand back and let me discover for myself what my limitations might be.

Many years later, my mother admitted that there were often times when she watched fearfully from the kitchen window as I ran full tilt into a tree or backyard fence. She fought the natural impulse to rush out to the rescue unless I really seemed hurt. She held her breath as I climbed trees, stood on the seat to pump my swing, or played rough and tumble games with my younger brothers. Sometimes, she put aside housework to help me learn to roller skate or jump rope. Never did she impose her own fears for my safety on me. She always encouraged me to try new things, understanding that this was the only way I would learn to handle them. She didn't want her fear transmitted to me, burdening me with another handicap to overcome, in addition to blindness.

As I grew into a young girl, she taught me how to do housework, sew, and cook. This not only gave her an extra pair of hands around the house but permitted me a sense of competence and usefulness. I never realized that the reason she directed me from another room through the steps of preparing a meal was because she found it difficult to watch me handling sharp knives or hot pans on the stove or in the oven.

She worked hard to see that I didn't develop any of the "blindisms" that would single me out as different from my sighted peers. She gently admonished me to look in her direction when I spoke to her and to hold my head up high. She offered advice on which colors went together and looked best on me. She spent a lot of time shopping and sewing for me to make sure I dressed in the latest fashions. She taught me to feel confidence in my appearance and to take pride in good grooming.

She drove miles to take me to special camps and other activities with visually impaired youngsters, so that I could practice such social skills as learning to dance. I could then take these skills and use them confidently back in my sighted community. Most of all, my mother gave me the gift of freedom to try my wings. She held back from offering me comfort when I fell unless I was actually hurt, gave it freely when I was, and never intimated that she thought I might fall. My wonderful mom understood that to truly love a handicapped child meant that she must suffer in silence through her own fears and doubts and let me go. She knew instinctively that if she tried to protect and shelter her little wounded chick, I might never learn to reach for my full potential in life.

I am now the mother of three grown children, grandmother of two, and married to a fine man, and I am a businesswoman. I was the first in my family to earn a college degree. I spent two and a half years serving in the Peace Corps and once climbed a 10,000-foot mountain. All of these accomplishments are mine because my mother was brave enough to let me run and play, to explore and grow, just like her other four unimpaired children. She was always there to offer a hug or word of encouragement but never there to teach me her fears. She was the wind beneath my wings.

Reprinted with permission from DeAnna Quietwater Noriega and *The Braille Forum*, volume 36, number 11, May 1998.

We find this particularly inspiring account of a blind woman's early life especially intriguing.

Next is the testimony of Ann Morris Bliss, founder and formerly chief executive officer of Ann Morris Enterprises Inc., a mail-order company that distributes products for the blind. Mrs. Bliss is a strong, capable, modern businesswoman and entrepreneur, the original inspiration for this book.

She has written about her early life:

I had low vision from birth until age 19, when I lost my residual vision. I raised two children mostly as a single parent and traveled with both a guide dog and a white cane.

In 1986 I began my mail-order company with one product and ended with over 1,000 when I sold it in 2004. I produced an annual catalog in large print, cassette, Braille, and electronic format and distributed over 50,000 copies yearly. Much time was spent traveling throughout the country selling items and helping others at organized conventions for the blind as well as local meetings and seminars. I was often consulted on starting and maintaining a successful business as well as researching and producing needed products to benefit visually impaired persons. My focus is now on spiritual healing and inner peace.

Here is her message to anyone coping with vision loss:

## THE ART OF LIVING WITH VISION LOSS
### *by Ann Morris Bliss*

My hope is that the next few pages will bring you comfort in knowing that vision loss is perfectly manageable. You may use some of the suggestions below as a starting point for using your own resourcefulness and ingenuity for success. Having a positive outlook is paramount to achieving a wholesome life. The power of intent is very important to success. When you fully know that you can conquer any obstacles in your path, they will be conquered. When you fully realize that you are a special person, your mind will be at ease. When you see your new life as an adventure, you will overcome. Vision loss will expand your other senses if you allow it. It will open the opportunity to really listen to others and to observe from a totally different prospective. I encourage you to embrace the new you and see how wondrous life can be.

Before I begin, I would like to briefly explain why I feel qualified to write this excerpt. I was a premature baby placed in an incubator. An incorrect amount of oxygen caused my vision loss. I had very poor vision throughout school. I wore very thick magnifying lenses for reading and had very little distance vision. Even if I sat in the first row, I could not read what was written on the blackboard. At age 16, my left eye failed, and at 19 I became totally unseeing. During the next 37 years I married, raised two beautiful and intelligent daughters, held several jobs, and owned and operated a mail-order catalog company specializing in items for persons with vision loss. I had no difficulty cooking, cleaning, sewing, using a computer, swimming, walking, and leading a very productive life. You too can do all of this and more ... much, much more.

Let me begin by saying that the Internet is an invaluable resource for finding solutions and information. If you do not use the Internet or know someone who does, your local library can help. Search engines such as Google or Yahoo! can be used for finding rehabilitation services, social services, low-vision specialists, and support groups in your area. You can find articles on accomplishing any task with little or no vision and use this invaluable tool for purchasing those needed aids and devices especially produced for functioning with vision loss. The resources listed at the end of this chapter may be useful for further investigation and purchase. An information hotline answers just about any question related to your daily living queries and governmental assistance. Use these resources and don't hesitate to ask the questions over and over until you receive the information you require.

Low-vision specialists are the best source for fitting you with lenses and magnification devices to make the most of your remaining useful residual vision. They can provide handheld magnifiers, magnifying lenses, telescopic lenses, monoculars and binoculars, and much more. Be sure to ask them about specific lighting to enhance your new low-vision devices. They may advise you on how to perform eye exercises such as those of the Bates Method to strengthen and enhance your vision. Consult these specialists often as your vision changes. Some areas have low-vision stores where you can actually try out additional magnifiers. Mail order offers a wide selection of items, and you can return an item if it's not appropriate.

Devices commonly known as closed-circuit televisions are cameras and monitors that magnify a paper, an object, or a book up to 65 times, in color or black and white, on a dark or light background, onto a television or separate monitor or screen. Company representatives will bring these right to your home for evaluation.

The Library of Congress provides a talking book program through which any legally blind person may borrow, at no cost, from their collection of 65,000 recorded books. The cost of special playback equipment as well as the books and magazines is funded by the U.S. government. The books are professionally narrated and can provide a lifetime of enjoyment. There are even national sports and news magazines. The program offers video and DVD movies that have a built-in track with audio explanations of what is occurring in the movie.

Local public libraries offer books printed in large type as well as books recorded on CDs and cassettes. A free service allows you to listen to hundreds of newspaper articles and television listings read every day through synthesized speech over your telephone. In many areas, radio-reading-service volunteers read news articles, local grocery ads, and items of interest over a separate sub-carrier or on a secondary audio programming channel on your television. Large-button and talking remote controls simplify channel changing for many. Many movie theaters throughout our country offer headphones so you can listen to the special audio track that explains the action. Local theatrical companies often also provide this wonderful service.

Navigating around your home and outdoors can be a challenge. Rehabilita-tion services provide mobility and orientation training at your residence and place of employment. They can determine if you are a candidate for a long white cane or a guide dog. In the meantime, you can learn your surroundings by no-ticing the different textures of carpets and flooring, different lighting, different smells, and the sounds of different spaces. Putting your hand in front of your body and horizontal to it will enable you to avoid obstacles and walls. Walk slowly until you learn a layout, and count steps if it is helpful. Textured tape or door mats may be put in front of stairs or other tricky areas. Use whatever lights make navigation easier. Guide ropes or patio blocks or rubber mats can often be used on your property to guide you from a doorway to a clothes line, seating area, or swimming pool.

Reflective tape strips can be an invaluable aid in dark areas, protecting you from being hit by motorists, pedestrians, or bicyclists.

When using public transportation, ask the driver to either announce the stops or advise you when your stop is reached. Most areas have a paratransit system. This is a door-to-door van service that will take you to doctors' offices, shopping, senior citizen centers, or to a friend, depending on the level of service in your area. Try calling your town hall and asking for the office for the handi-capped. You can make a sign to hold up that says TAXI for flagging one down. Airlines are wonderful at assisting you on and off your flight as well as guid-ing you to your connecting flight and to baggage claim. Never hesitate to ask for assistance. Lapel pins that state "I have low vision" are available to notify the public that you may require some special service. Even if you don't actually use a white cane, you might consider holding one as a comfort while asking for help.

When walking with a sighted guide, it is customary to walk slightly behind and with your hand on the back of the guide's arm. With a little practice you will be able to feel the direction the guide is walking and whether there are steps. Pamphlets on guiding a visually impaired person are available.

Conversing with loved ones and friends is even more important now. Most phone companies have special-needs phones and services, so call and inquire about them. With practice, you can learn to dial the phone accurately, or you can use operator assistance. Voice-activated phones and dialers are available as well as phones with very large numbers and buttons. Cell phone magnifiers may also be helpful. Your phone company may also have special large-print overlays for your phone at no charge.

Labeling items and being especially organized in your home will be particularly important now. If you can see what you are writing, check out your stationery store for a great selection of Sharpies, Expresso 20/20 pens, and more as well as different point thicknesses. Paper with widely spaced heavy black lines is available. Envelope, letter writing, and signature guides aid in writing straight and in the proper location. Check-writing guides and large-print check registers are available Your bank can furnish large-print checks or checks that have raised lines and are oversize. Most banks have automated services for you to use to ascertain your balance, which checks have cleared, and which deposits have been recorded. Ask your bank to provide a large-print or Braille statement, and if they cannot, ask for someone to read it to you each month.

Talking Rx is a chip that can be attached to prescription bottles. The chips can be programmed by your pharmacist or anyone else to audibly tell you the medication and the dosage. Inquire at your pharmacy or through one of the aids and devices catalogs. Bottles may be differentiated by using different colored tape, rubber bands, size, or location on your shelf or table. Create a system and stick to it. A handheld tape recorder may be useful for recording your system as well as recording phone numbers and notes. Different tapes may be used for unique purposes, such as one for phone numbers, one for recipes, and one for notes. Large tactile dots are very helpful for differentiating tapes, marking switches, and labeling appliances. They are available in many sizes and colors.

If you can no longer identify the colors of your clothing, oversize safety pins with large, molded dots can be placed on the inside of the care label or pinned inside a hem. Just create a system as to which pin configuration represents which color. Often alphabetical order helps in remembering your system. Talking color identifiers tell you the solid color of an item and are very useful in matching clothes, socks, and shoes. A talking bar code reader enables you to create a label on which you can record the color as well as any other pertinent information. These labels can be sewn on, adhered to, or rubber-banded around an item. Possible uses include clothing, medications, CDs, folders, tapes, spices, cleansers, and cans. Some are so sophisticated that they will tell you the contents of a can or package of food or drink by its bar code. There are so many wonderful products available to solve almost any quandary.

Specially designed wallets often contain many compartments for separating paper currency, or you may choose to use your existing wallet and fold each bill in a certain way. Coin pouches enable you to sort your coins. One clue is that dimes and quarters have serrated edges than can be felt with your fingernail.

You may want to purchase a paper-money identifier, which tells you the denomination of each bill, for added security.

The microwave oven is a wonderful invention and can be marked with tactile or colored dots if you do not choose a talking unit. They provide little excuse for not eating. Take a friend to the supermarket to explore your options for microwave cooking. Stoves and other appliances may be marked with dots, and different colors and overlays may be available; consult the manufacturer. When shopping for a new appliance, consult the blindness consumer groups for suggestions of current models that comply with Americans with Disabilities Act (ADA) standards. Safety should be your main concern while cooking, but any task can be done with little or no vision. A cooking show for the visually impaired is available on the Internet.

The key to a clean surface is to create an overlapping grid so that all areas will be covered. This works for vacuuming, mopping, and cleaning counters and tubs. Remember, there is a solution to every worry, and it may be as easy as a phone call to one of the numbers listed below. Let these resources and the personnel behind them work for you, and in turn, you may be able to pass the information along to others.

Ann Morris Bliss gives much good and helpful advice stemming from her years as a teacher at the Institute for the Blind and her personal experience as a blind woman navigating in the world independently. Story reprinted with permission.

## TRAGEDY TRANSFORMED TO HEALTH, PURPOSE, AND A NEW CAREER

### *by Melissa Moody, CMT*

In 1992 I was run over by an SUV in Texas and nearly killed. Massive injuries included a crushed face, brain injury, broken ribs, punctured lung, double vision, and many musculoskeletal problems. My struggles were compounded by a rear-end collision four years later, in which I suffered a ruptured disc and a herniated disc in my neck. In 1997, after years of physical therapy and more than 26 reconstructive surgeries, I still suffered constant chronic pain, limited movement, and double vision.

It was then I read *Self-Healing, My Life and Vision* by Meir Schneider, PhD, LMT, and hope stirred within me. Meir is a health care pioneer and visionary who overcame his own blindness and has facilitated the successful recovery of innumerable others. I resolved to get to San Francisco and the School for Self-Healing to see if he could help me. Initially I went because I had lost what little binocular vision strabismus surgery had given me. (I had a type of tunnel vision in which I could see one image while looking straight ahead, but even with the surgery, everything was double in my peripheral vision and in any direction other than directly in front of me.) Ophthalmic specialists were puzzled and offered no solution. Constant double vision is disorienting, like living in a moving kaleidoscope. In the fall of 1997 I traveled to San Francisco for two weeks of therapy with Meir. I regained the recently lost fusion noninvasively, but even more surprising to me, I suffered less pain in my body and could move more freely. I went home armed with hope and my home program.

After a couple of more visits, Meir suggested I take his Self-Healing Segment A class to better understand how to continue to work on myself. I thought I was too disabled to undertake such an endeavor, but he encouraged me and thought it would really help. Completing the class transformed my life. Immersing myself for 10 days allowed me to internalize the principles as well as experience dramatic change and improvement. Thrilled with the improvements I made and intrigued with the effectiveness of self-healing, I approached the Texas Rehabilitation Commission (TRC) to ask if it would underwrite further classes. But after a vocational evaluation, TRC declined, deeming me too disabled. Undeterred, I found other support and resources through family and friends.

In 1999 I underwent an orbital (eye socket) reconstruction surgery in Seattle and suffered postoperative complications that nearly blinded me in my right eye. After a month in Seattle, I moved to San Francisco to work intensively with Meir and cornea specialists at the University of California at San Francisco Medical Center. After about six months the specialists had eliminated a corneal infection and done all they could. I continued working with Meir on my vision and my recovery for the rest of my body. In gratitude, I started volunteering at the school, and in 2001 I started working part-time at the school, the first time I'd been able to work in nearly 10 years!

As I grew stronger, I increased my hours. Even the residual effects of my brain injury improved. In 2003 I became the education and development director at the School for Self-Healing. In 2004 I passed the Department of Motor Vehicles vision test and received my unrestricted California driver's license! I am a Self-Healing practitioner and a natural vision improvement educator. I love being able to help others now.

Except for minor disfigurement in my face, no one would have a clue of what I have been through. And I unreservedly engage in favorite activities like gardening and cooking, impossible a few years ago. Whereas in 1999 I could not even plan a dinner party and I was in so much chronic pain I could not hold a garden hose for more than five minutes at a time, today I freely garden, dance, and so on, and in the fall of 2004 I organized my exquisite wedding for 100 people! I am a walking miracle, trauma transcended and transformed. It has taken patience, motivation, and work, but I never dreamed the quality of my life could be what it is today. You can improve, too!

Reprinted with permission from Melissa Moody.

The author of the next true story is Mack Riley, a popular teacher at the Braille Institute's Los Angeles Center.

## THE JOY OF PARENTING: SINGLE, BLIND, WORKING FATHER TAKES CARE OF FIVE-YEAR-OLD SON

### *by Mack Riley*

When sighted people find out that I am a single father, they don't ask how I take care of my five-year-old son, but who takes care of him. This is even before they learn that I am an employed teacher. The questions people ask upon becoming aware that my son and I live in a four-room flat without benefit of a mother, grandparents, or live-in help include "Who prepares your meals?" "Who takes your son to school?" "Who helps your son with his homework?" I tell the woman sitting next to us on the bus that we had cereal, eggs, toast, melon, and juice for breakfast, and that it was I who prepared it before getting Jonathan ready for school. We are on our way to school now. When I drop him off, I will catch another bus and go to my job as a teacher at the Braille Institute.

The woman is puzzled. She wonders aloud, "How can you see to teach?"

I smile, facing her. "I cannot see you even though I am two feet from you," I try to explain.

"You mean you don't know what your son looks like?" she asks sadly.

I explain to her that I do know what my son looks like, even though I have never seen him visually. "I know the shape of his nose, the curve of his mouth, the size and shape of his ears, the texture of his hair, the shape of his chin, his attitude, the color of his hair and his eyes, and even the little bump on the bottom of his foot which was caused by stepping on a tack."

We get off the bus at our stop.

My son holds on to my hand as we negotiate the crumbling, narrow sidewalk to his school. There are children at the gate, waiting. Some of them call out my son's name. The little children guide me through the gate as my son disappears among them. They laugh. They do not ask me about my blindness. They do not doubt that I am Jonathan's father. They do not ask me how I take care of him.

I return through the gate and walk two blocks to a bus stop where I board the bus to go to my own school, where I teach. Even though I hold two degrees and three California teaching credentials for life that among them have permitted me to teach preschool through community college, I am often viewed as incapable by casual observers.

I don't mean to suggest that losing one's sight does not present problems. As matter of fact, suddenly finding oneself blind can be as traumatic as losing a loved one, but it can be overcome, as exemplified by many active blind persons who sought appropriate training and re-adaptation of skills.

At the Braille Institute in Los Angeles, I teach newly blind people skills for daily living. I think I often jostle the minds of my students, especially those who arrive in my classroom with a helpless and hopeless attitude. I jostle their minds into a more accepting attitude toward their visual loss when I tell them that, as a single father, I take care of my five-year-old son, take him to school before I come to work, prepare our meals, and still make time to help him learn (I taught him kindergarten in two months). I also make time to write a few pages in either of my journals or on one of my ongoing projects: short stories, biographies, family history, poems, or articles for magazines.

After I have greeted a new student at the door and walked about the room during the class session, I then tell him or her I am also blind. More than one student has challenged me on this, saying, "You must be a high partial." I have only a sliver of light perception in one eye. It is at this time that I tell how I once was unbelieving also. I never fail to mention the blind auto mechanic, the blind lawyer, and the blind ballet dancer. I tell them that they are not abnormal by feeling this way at this point as a newly blind person. I felt that way, too. In this way, I am perhaps one of the most credible teachers at the Braille Institute. I am particularly proud of the example I am living as a single, blind, working father of a five-year-old. My son is totally in my care. In that way, I am unique. My son and I, in addition to going to school and work every day, go walking in the neighborhood, take a bus shopping, and go to church on Sunday, and on Independence Day we took a picnic lunch to Griffith Park. I don't depend on him to guide me, although one day when we were looking for an electronics shop, he insisted that it was the next door after the one I was about to enter. When we got inside, I discovered that he had guided me into a toy store.

My son and I get along together just great. Every day before and after dinner, we can be found on the floor playing with toy cars; at the breakfast table, working on new vocabulary, phonetics, and spelling; at any time, playing hide 'n' seek; or at bedtime, telling each other fairytales or me teaching him Mother Goose rhymes.

Sometimes I think I am trying to make up for lost time with him. We were separated for more than three years when he was abducted. I spent three long years looking for him, first finding him in New Zealand and then having to start all over when he disappeared and then was found in the United States. I became a fairly good detective and learned a great deal about child custody laws. Three long years, court battles, and the efforts of detectives, lawyers, judges, the U.S. department of state, the New Zealand government, law officials, and friends finally resulted in the two of us being reunited. It was not easy in the beginning, for Jonathan did not know his real name. However, now all that is in the past, and a bright future looms ahead. I can imagine the sun brightly glistening in his yellow hair and his blue eyes, like the sky on a clear day, and him turning up to me and saying, "Show me the way, Daddy."

I do, and we walk the full way into the future together.

With him, I forget I am blind.

Story courtesy of Mack Riley. Reprinted with permission from Lea Seelig Riley.

The following account, divided into chapters, was written by a young woman, Betsy Coffman Grenevitch, originally from West Virginia. It tells in full detail about her life growing up and her Christian faith, attending the School for the Blind and eventually Fairmont State University in Fairmont, West Virginia.

After a physical description of her foster home in West Virginia, where she was raised because her young birth mother was unable to care for her, Betsy describes the engaging menagerie in her home.

## IS THIS A ZOO OR A FARM?

We lived about seven miles from town. Our house was on a dirt road along with a barn, shed, pigpen, chicken house, and another house right beside the main road. As far back as I can remember, we always had animals that you could expect to have on a farm: sheep, goats, cows, pigs, ponies, chickens, ducks, geese, turkeys, dogs, and cats. But we also had many other kinds of animals, some of which I will tell you about now. For example, let me tell you the story of Ginger.

### Ginger, the Baby Goat

Ginger was born in the winter. Her mother died at her birth; we brought her to the house so that she would not die. We fed her with a bottle, and we rocked her to sleep. We used a bread bag for a diaper. How many people do you know who kept a baby goat in their house?

### Rachel, the Raccoon

We kept not only farm animals but also wild animals. I was especially fond of Rachel, our pet raccoon. When she was a baby, we would lead her around on a leash and let her climb the pear tree that was in the front yard. Dad also built a cage for her and put a tree stump in it. From the beginning, Rachel liked bread and jelly, cookies, cereal, and peanuts. Before eating the peanuts, she would wipe off all the salt with her fingers. Sometimes we would let her eat in the house. When she did, she would eat in the high chair. Many times we gave her a sardine can with cereal and another can with water because raccoons wash their food before they eat it.

In the summer we would sit on the glider on the side porch, and Rachel would play with our hair and nibble at our ears. She would also climb up and down our backs. Rachel acted very much like a little child. When no one was looking, she would get into trouble. One time she wandered up the back stairs and found a marble game. She started rolling the marbles down the stairs and then carried them back up again. Rachel also had another place she liked to go when no one was looking. We kept our eggs on top of the freezer in egg cartons, and she liked to take them out and play ball with them. Rachel ran away once, but after several months she returned and was with us for the remainder of her life.

### Bambi

She was a baby deer and should have been called Faline, but I guess whoever named her got the names a little mixed up. Someone found her along the road and did not see her mother anywhere; so he brought her to us.

She was treated like a queen when she was growing up. We fed her with a bottle until she was old enough to eat off a plate. She stood between Mom and Dad and ate off a plate right on the table. Believe it or not, she never made a mess! She ate the same food we did. She especially loved ice cream!

When she was small, she would sleep in the bathtub during the daytime. At night she would sleep on a rug by Mom and Dad's bed. When she had to use the bathroom, Mom would hear her get up and would put a little baby potty under her.

Below is a newspaper article written at the time about Bambi.

### PET DEER

"The Coffman household in Antioch has a pet deer which even has its own place at the dining table between Herb and Elizabeth. The Coffmans have four children around the house to pamper Bambi, the deer. Now five months old, Bambi has a new outfit—a red shirt and a red collar and bell. When asked if it was Bambi's Christmas outfit, Mrs. Coffman said it was to protect Bambi from hunters in the Antioch area. Bambi stays in the house quite a bit though." (*The Mineral Daily*)

### Mitsy

We also kept some dogs in the house. My sister got Mitsy after she was married, and somehow we ended up with her. She, along with a cat, slept with me, and they were good company. When I was feeling sad, I would often go and find Mitsy and talk to her and lay my head on her and cry. Sometimes I really thought she understood what I was saying by the way she licked me. We had a lot of good times together....

During that same week I had interviews with the director of admissions, dean of fine arts, and dean of education [at Bob Jones University]. I was the first blind person to apply for their education degree program. During one interview, one of the men asked me how I was going to teach sighted children. When I heard these words, I determined in my heart that I would prove to them that a blind person could teach as well as anyone else, with very minor adjustments.

I received word shortly after these interviews that I was accepted as a student at Bob Jones University....

## ROUGH EDGES—REACTIONS AND RESPONSES

I still have rough edges that need to be polished, and some that will probably never be as smooth as I would like, but in spite of my imperfections, my heavenly Father still loves me and wants to use me.

In this chapter, I want to share with you some examples of these rough edges. Some of these may appear only in the life of a blind person, but that still does not give him/her the excuse to keep repeating the same mistakes.

Outspokenness. Many blind people say just what they think. Often their outspokenness results in hurt feelings. I have done this many times without ever knowing it because I cannot see the expression on the other person's face.

When a sighted person makes this mistake, he has the advantage of seeing the other person and is able to apologize immediately. Many times I have not learned about the hurt I caused for several weeks. Often another person would tell me what they had heard from the person I had hurt. Sometimes I said something in a joking manner that was taken seriously. When I asked why people would not tell me right then that I had hurt them, my friends would say that they were afraid to say anything. I told them that I was hurt more by their telling someone else than if they had just told me.

"I Can Do It!" Many times when I was around new people, I would not let them help me because I wanted to show them that I could do things for myself. If I could not do something, I would just do without it. An example of my doing without concerns cutting up meat. For the Sunday noon meal at Bob Jones, we would often have ham. Because it was so difficult for me to cut, I would just do without it.

After doing that for several months, I finally relented, and let someone cut it for me. Another example of my wanting to do something on my own concerned crossing the streets. At Bob Jones University, the drivers have the right-of-way, which can be very dangerous for a blind person. One day during my second semester, I was going to literature class. Many students were walking in the same direction as I was and were talking; so it was difficult for me to hear if there were any cars coming. I was also at a street that is near the fountains, which made it even harder to hear. I had stopped to listen and did not hear any-thing; so I started across the street. The next thing I knew, my knees collided with a moving object. The only thing that kept me from falling was my cane. Physically I was not hurt, but I could not believe that no one nearby had tried to warn me that an electric cart was coming.

Even when I would let someone help me, I found out that he would often try to beat an approaching car and I was not willing to do that—especially after being hit. I would not cross unless I could not hear a car, no matter how far away it was. I have this big fear only at the university, since everywhere else I travel pedestrians have the right-of-way and the drivers are watching out for me. Even now, several years after the incident, I am still very much afraid when crossing streets at the university with or without another person.

When people would try to help me across the street, sometimes I would an-swer in the wrong way, especially if I had been asked many times that day. Some-times I would say, "I can do it OK," or "I'd rather do it on my own." I did not find out until much later that in the South if I did not put "thank you" in my response somewhere, I was being rather rude. I also found out that I was offending many people just because I would not let them help me. As time went on, I became more and more frustrated. One day I had the opportunity to talk about this prob-lem with one of my professors. I explained to him that one of the reasons I wanted to cross on my own was that I needed to keep depending on my ears and not the eyes of others. He said that I was right because there would be times when there would not be anyone around to help me and if I became too dependent on people, I would not be able to cross on my own. [Here Betsy Coffman details the questions any blind person is frequently asked and gives her answers to them.]

Questions: I am tired of the ridiculous ones. I realize now that people ask questions because they are not familiar with the situation, but up until 1983, I did not think of it that way. Here are some examples of questions that were the hardest for me.

1. Do your roommates help you get dressed?
2. How do you find your mouth when you are eating?
3. Do you count your steps when you walk?
4. Don't you have better hearing than I do?
5. Your memory is better than mine, isn't it?
6. I don't have to hold onto you when we're walking so you won't fall?
7. You have perfect pitch since you're blind, don't you?

8. Aren't all blind people the same in what they can and cannot do?
9. How do I talk to a blind person? I'm afraid I'll say the wrong things.
10. How do I know when to help a blind person? I'm tired of hearing, "I don't need your help."

In case some of you have wondered about these questions but never asked anyone about them, let me answer them for you.

1. My roommates did not help me get dressed! When you cannot see, your fingers become your eyes and you can feel by the shape of the garment which way it goes on.
2. Do you look at your mouth with a mirror while you are eating? No, of course not. It is something that each one of us just learns naturally. Not long ago I heard a good response to this question given by Fanny Crosby, talking about eating while at the blind school. "They tie a string to the leg of the table and the other end to my mouth. I just slide the spoon up the string to find my mouth."
3. Counting my steps while walking would get rather boring. Then I also would not be able to carry on a conversation with anyone. Most blind people learn after several times of trial and error how to judge the distance from one point to the next.
4. My hearing is not better than yours. I have just had to develop that sense to help replace my eyes. It does not happen without working on it.
5. I was not born with a better memory than yours. In fact, many of you have better memories than I do.
6. If I hold on to you in the correct manner and you walk naturally, I will not fall. The sighted person should keep the arm that the blind person is holding straight down. The blind person who has been trained will automatically hold on to your elbow and will try to stay a step behind you. Just because a person cannot see does not mean that he cannot walk. If the above procedures are followed, you will find yourself forgetting that the person cannot see.
7. For years, people have thought that all blind people are musically inclined and have perfect pitch. I can assure you that this is false because I do not have perfect pitch and must work on music just as many of you do.
8. Can all sighted people do the same things? The same goes for those who are blind. Some of us are more adventurous than others and are willing to try anything. Some of us accept challenges; some run from them.

9. The first time I was really exposed to this question was at a youth conference at Hyles-Anderson College. I began to notice that people were
   talking to my friends but not to me. I could not understand why. I had
   been taking notes at the meetings, and one day a young person asked
   me to show her how I did it. In the midst of our conversation, I found
   out why people were not talking to me. They thought they had to talk
   to me in a different manner and were afraid they would not do it right.
   For example, they were afraid to use the words see, watch, or look at.
   A blind person uses the same vocabulary as everyone else. For example, I would say to a friend "I saw Larry this morning." It would not
   sound right if I said I heard or touched Larry this morning because people don't talk that way. [Her advice:] Please talk to a blind person the
   same way you would talk to a sighted friend.

10. My response to this question is simple. If you do not know the blind
   person, do not offer your assistance unless you are absolutely certain
   that he needs it. Then you will not be told "no" again, and the blind
   person will not feel like a child.

I do not need—nor do I want—your pity! I have felt this way so many times
that I cannot count them. By the way a person talks to me, I can tell if he is pity-
ing me. I have also found out through the years that this is the motive of many
people who offer their help. They like to go and tell their friends about helping
"the blind girl" today. It has been hard for me to let some strangers help me because I feel they do it for the wrong reasons. But I am trying not to let it bother
me, and I do let people help me more than I did in the past—but not all the time
as I still need to be independent as much as possible.

[Some exclaim,] You don't know me! How many of you recognize every person that you have met only once before the very next time you meet them? I can
recall many times when someone would come up to me and say, "Hi! Don't you
remember me?" When I would say that I did not, they would say, "But I met
you yesterday!" Sometimes I would become frustrated and reply, "Many people
speak to me, and I cannot remember all their names and their voices."

[Or some ask,] Why aren't you smiling today? I became very angry after being
asked this question many times in one day. Inside I was screaming, "Can't I
have a normal life which includes both bad and good days? Do I always have to
be smiling just to please others? Folks, I'm just like you! I'm normal!"

I'm tired of everyone watching me! This was one of my biggest struggles
while attending Bob Jones University. Quite often, I would have people tell me
that they had been watching me and were fascinated by all I was able to do.
Others would say that they were watching me and that I was a big encouragement to them. I started thinking, "Can't I go anywhere and not have so many

people watching me? I want to go and hide from everyone. If I were not blind, I could be normal and not constantly be observed by thousands of people!"

[Some say,] If I were blind, I could never do what you are doing. False! You cannot say what you could or could not do unless you were in the situation. As I have already mentioned, a blind person learns to develop other senses to replace the eyes. Please do not put a blind person on a pedestal. You can do what you have to do when the time comes. Where there is a will, there is a way.

[When asked about her cane, she says,] It's only a cane! This incident took place several times while I attended Bob Jones University, but in different versions. When I walked alone, I always used my cane because it helped me to walk much faster. Most of the time I could hear if someone was in front of me, and if there was, I would slow down to avoid hitting them. However, when walking on carpet, I could not tell if there was anyone in front of me unless he were talking. That was the case when the following incident took place. I was walking out of the dorm lobby when my cane hit a foot. All of a sudden a girl screamed and asked the monitor to get the dog out of there as she was afraid of them. After she went out the door, we started laughing. When I got outside and she saw what had really happened, she was embarrassed. Even though I was frustrated because of what happened, I had to admit that it was quite funny.

Some of these rough edges will never become as smooth as I would like, but remember, I am striving to do my best, with God's grace, to smooth them as much as possible. If I have offended any of you, please forgive me....

### EPILOGUE

This [writing] . . . was first started in March, 1987. I thought it would be nice to bring you up to date on my whereabouts now.

I married Larry Grenevitch in August 1988. We have four children: Danielle Joy, 13, Paul George, 10, Joshua Dallas, 6, and Michelle Kay, 2.

## IN THE LIONS CAMP: A MEMOIR

### *by Douglas M. Karlen*

From the map room of memory, I can still call up the camp layout. Now, more than four decades after my time there, I can still imagine it all—the bluff overlooking the lake; the dining hall atop the bluff; the flagpole out in front; the office and staff dormitory across the gravel driveway; the arts and crafts cabin close by; the girls' cabins off in the distance; the boys' cabins straight down the steep hill; the lake nearby, with its small sand beach and short wooden pier; and the wilderness beyond the beach. The camp seems huge in memory. In reality, it was not—just the land surrounding the lake.

It was a small lake. One could hike completely around the lake in about an hour, traversing through several different ecosystems in the process. First, just beyond the beach, the hiker had to pass through a forest where he or she was sure to trip over roots and fallen limbs. Then, turning (in what direction I cannot remember), the hiker had to slog through a marsh where he or she was likely to get mud on his or her shoes. Then, on the far side of the lake, the hiker had to wade through prairie grass. The bugs were thickest in the grassland, but the hiker could at least get the mud off his or her shoes here before returning to civilization. Finally, the hiker had to climb the bluff (a much easier climb on this far side than the steep ascent from the boys' cabins), pass the girls' cabins, and stop at the dining hall for a refreshing glass of Kool-Aid. We campers trekked around the lake several times, but we never went alone. We always had our counselors to guide us.

I can imagine it now; I had to imagine it then, too. I did not see it then; or, at least, I did not see it well. Few of the campers saw it. This was the Lions Camp for children who were blind or visually impaired. The Lions Club owned and operated this camp near Rosholt, Wisconsin. For one week every summer, the Wisconsin Lions opened the camp to kids sponsored by Illinois Lions Clubs. Through the efforts of my parents and teachers and the sponsorship of the Mont Clare Lions, I was lucky enough to go to camp for one week each August in three consecutive years—1958, 1959, and 1960.

Memories of incidents and details from those distant years have melted together. It is difficult to distinguish one camp trip from another. Therefore, unless noted otherwise, this memoir will treat all of my camp experiences as a single journey. The feelings generated by that journey, on the other hand, are easy to recall. They were good feelings.

* * *

Getting to camp was half the fun—at least for the first two years. With my camp things neatly packed into a small suitcase, my father drove me downtown to the old Greyhound Bus Station at Clark and Randolph. Mom went along too, to wish me a good trip and to make sure I boarded the right bus. Because there was no space for a terminal on the busy streets in the Loop, buses loaded and unloaded underground at the old station. Departing passengers took escalators down to the departure area below street level. For me, the departure area was always a mass of confusion—suitcases strewn everywhere, kids wandering or crying (sometimes both), parents yelling or crying (sometimes both), incomprehensible announcements over the loudspeakers, annoyed passengers trying to go somewhere other than to camp, and so on. Fortunately, there were always enough cool-headed parents and Lions volunteers to sort things out properly. Somehow, we campers all got on the right bus, shepherded through glass departure doorways marked with gate numbers only the adults could see. I settled in for the long ride, peering out the tinted windows. There was little to see at first—just the blank walls of the tunnel that led from the station to the outside world. Then, as we emerged into daylight, I could see the Chicago River, then city streets, then highways, and, ultimately, open country. I may have slept a little, too.

We stopped for lunch in Fond du Lac, Wisconsin. As the name suggests (although I did not know it at the time), this small town is located at the southern tip of a lake—Lake Winnebago. We stopped at a park on the lakeshore, and the local Lions Club served us a fantastic lunch. The Lions might have grilled up hot dogs or hamburgers. I do not remember the main course; I do remember the corn on the cob. It was the best sweet corn ever. I have never tasted better. I shall never forget the joy of that corn on the cob, and I have remembered it in all the years since whenever I am eating (enjoying, even) a pale substitute.

After lunch, we clambered aboard the bus again and completed our journey to camp. We missed all this excitement on my third camp trip. We took a train from Chicago Union Station to Stevens Point, Wisconsin, and then bussed the final 20 minutes or so to camp. Alas, no Fond du Lac lunch; no Fond du Lac corn!

Upon our arrival in camp, we formed up around the flagpole and received our cabin assignments. We would be engaging in most camp activities as a group with our cabin mates, so cabin assignment was important. You did not want to be stuck with bullies or babies in your cabin. The counselors—college men and women probably majoring in education or social work—lined us up in our assigned groups. The girls then scampered off to their nearby cabins. We boys struggled down the steep hill with our suitcases.

Your cabin mates mattered; the actual cabin did not. All the cabins were alike—equally disappointing. At the bottom of the hill, we found our cabin to be the simplest of shelters—a square wooden frame structure with bare concrete floors. Cots were lined up along the four walls. Other than a phone on the wall near the door, there were no interior decorations or other furnishings. There was no bathroom, either.

"Outhouse," our counselor explained, "out the door and to your left. There's a washhouse [sinks and showers but no toilets] down near the beach. That's it, boys. This is the wilderness!"

He was right about that. It was primitive. You could not even dial the phone. It was an old fashioned crank phone. If you cranked the handle, every phone on the party line would ring. Each cabin (and, I presume, the office and staff dorm) was on the party line and had a signal code—two short rings and a long, for example. With a system like that, one thing was clear. We could not phone home. We were here for the duration. That was fine with me.

As our counselor supervised our settling-in process, I chose a bed and unpacked my camp things. Mom had packed, carefully following the camp instruction sheet. I had my pajamas, towels, swim trunks, eyedrops, allergy pills, toothbrush, toothpaste, bug spray, suntan lotion, shirts, pants, and plenty of underwear. I was ready to rough it. Mom had sewn a label with my name on it into most of my things. Why? Who would read the label? Certainly not me or most of the other campers! We were blind or vision impaired. Perhaps my body was to be identified by the label in my underpants—just in case something happened to me. I put all my things in the drawer beneath my cot, filling up the only personal space we were allowed. With that, I was set for my camp experience.

\* \* \*

Camp days followed a routine. "Rise and Shine" came early with one annoying long ring of the cabin phone. After scrambling to use the outhouse and washhouse, we trudged up the hill to assemble at the flagpole. The girls were always at the flagpole first; they did not have to climb a hill. Once assembled, we stood at attention to recite the Pledge of Allegiance while the counselors raised the American flag. Then, it was on to breakfast. The rest of the morning was filled with arts and crafts, nature walks, and late-morning swimming. I was not a big fan of arts and crafts. I was not very good at it. Except for writing, typing, and piano playing (none being necessary camp skills), I was not good with my hands. My father, a very handy guy, never taught me how to do things with my hands or with tools. If he let me "assist" him on a project, he would do all the work—directing me to hold or fetch things while he hammered, sawed, or sanded. Why didn't he teach me or let me do the work? I don't know why. Whether he was merely acting on his own need to control every situation or whether he truly believed I was incapable, I do not know. In any event, I had no desire to make things. I always tried to see what I was doing rather than rely on touch. Because I did not see very well, things came out weird looking. So, in the arts and crafts cabin, I struggled with the plastic strips that had to be woven together to make lanyards or key chains and with the yarn that had to be stretched across a frame to make potholders. I was not proud of anything I made. I never brought any of it home. But, that was all right with me. I knew I would never be an artist or a craftsman. I knew I would be an intellectual. I knew I was going to college. I worried about some of my cabin mates, though—the ones who had less vision and less intellect than I. I knew that some people who are blind wind up earning a meager living in shops making things like key chains and potholders. Was the arts and crafts cabin simply a training ground, a practice session, for them? Would this be all they would ever achieve in life? It was sad to think that this might be all some people could get out of life. I hoped that all of our futures would be better than that.

After lunch, we enjoyed more hiking and swimming, as well as a brief nap period. One afternoon, we had a treasure hunt. Our counselor read clues to us, and we called out suggestions as to where in the camp we should look for the next clue or for the treasure itself. The treasure was not identified, but that did not matter. My cabin mates and I really wanted to find it, whatever it was. After searching through the entire camp—going from beach to forest to marsh to prairie and back again—we discovered the treasure on the shore in the marshland. We tugged on a rope and hauled out of the lake a gigantic watermelon. That was the treasure! As victors in the treasure hunt, my cabin mates and I won a reward; we received the first slices of the luscious melon.

Just before sunset each evening, all campers reassembled at the flagpole to lower the flag. The counselors showed us how to fold the flag into a neat, compact, triangular bundle. Then, it was on to dinner.

In the dining hall, we sat with our cabin mates at long tables. The food came to us family style—all the meat, all the vegetables, and so on heaped on a serving dish. Our counselor presided over our table, making sure each camper had plenty to eat and assisting those who needed help.

"Mashed potatoes at four o'clock," the counselor would say, hoping that his charges would keep their fingers out of the gravy while reaching for their utensils.

The food was good. Fortunately, either the cook never used nuts or peanuts or my counselor, forewarned of my food allergies, was watching out for me. I never had any problems with camp food. My mother, however, would have been shocked if she knew of one of the staples of our camp diet. We drank Kool-Aid all the time—gallons of it. "Bug Juice," our counselor called it as he filled our glasses with cherry Kool-Aid. "Yeah, we went out to the prairie on the other side of the lake and got these mosquitoes and . . ." We had a good laugh if a camper actually believed in Bug Juice.

After dinner, we sang. The girls seemed to enjoy the singing more than the boys, but we all joined in. We sang typical camp songs—simple tunes with repetitive lyrics. For example, one of our songs was

Rise and shine
And give God the glory, glory.
Rise and shine

And give God the glory, glory.
Rise and shine and [clap hands once]
Give God the glory, glory,
Children of the Lord.

This song occasionally degenerated into a shouting match between cabins. We were only slightly more musical with some of the other camp favorites—a song about a dog (or was it a horse?) named Bingo, something about a goat, a song about a guy named John Jacob Jingleheimer Smith, a song about Marching to Pretoria, and something about the city of "Amster-Amster-Dam-Dam-Dam." Here is my favorite camp lyric:

Do your ears hang low?
Do they wobble to and fro?
Can you tie 'em in a knot?
Can you tie 'em in a bow?
Can you throw them over your shoulder
Like a Continental soldier?
Do your ears hang low?

The singing over, we adjourned for the evening's real entertainment. In the darkness, we sat around a bonfire near the arts and crafts cabin. Sometimes, one of the older staff members dressed as an Indian chief and told Indian stories and ghost stories while we toasted marshmallows. The girls usually screamed at the ghost stories, especially at the climax of the classic "Who's Got My Golden Arm?" At other times, the same staffer, dressed as a clown, entertained us with jokes and riddles. As any good entertainer might, he pandered to his audience for participation and applause. He asked, "What's the difference between a comma and a cat?" No one knew. "A comma," he said, "is a pause at the end of a clause. A cat has claws at the end of his paws." (It's funnier when a clown says it than when a writer writes it.) Next, he asked, "If a plane crashes on the border of North Dakota and South Dakota, where do they bury the survivors?" Well, of course they don't bury the survivors anywhere; they're still alive! I knew that, but I usually kept quiet at these shows, preferring to enjoy the laughter and cheering but not to participate. Another time, he asked, "Do they have a Fourth of July in England?" Well, of course they do. "Sure," he said, "it's a day on their calendar, too." The final straw came one night when he asked how to pronounce the capital of Kentucky. He wanted to know, "Is it Loo-ee-vil, Loo-iss-vil, or Loo-uh-vil?" Everyone began shouting out their favorite choice—"Loo-ee-vil" predominating. This question and the raucous response overwhelmed my usual reticence, and my penchant for accuracy compelled me to speak.
      "Frankfort," I said. "The capital of Kentucky is Frankfort."

"Right you are," the clown said, tossing me a rubber hot dog—well, frank-furter, actually.

And so to bed. Nighttime was the true test of the Lions campers. We would be on our own. After "Lights Out," the counselors went off to do whatever college men and women do at night. They did not sleep in the cabins with their charges. They sent out night patrols every hour or so, shining flashlights through cabin windows. Other than that, however, we were on our own.

\* \* \*

If we had bullies or babies in our cabin, nighttime would give them the opportu-nity to display their character. Fortunately, we never had bullies. A bully had prob-ably victimized most of us campers at some time during our lives. In the eyes of the "normal" world, we campers were all unfortunate, all different, one way or another. "Normal" people, it seemed to me, never hesitated to point this out. Some, the bul-lies of the world, did this with malicious intent, hoping to gain some advantage—to extort money or to exercise power over someone too weak or too unwilling to ob-ject. Others, merely curious, just wanted to know what was wrong. I frequently suffered through a barrage of personal questions from strangers, questions such as "Did you forget your glasses?" or the classic "What's wrong with your eyes?" I never answered. I had no desire to tell total strangers my problems or my life story. Under questioning in this mode, I felt anger because the questioner made me feel as if I needed to explain, to justify, myself. I also felt pain because I knew, deep down, that my interrogator was right. I really did have a condition and an appearance that marked me as different or unfortunate, as a stranger might put it. I often felt like crying when I heard these questions. In any event, whether it was harassment or merely a thoughtless question, I hated any reminder of my handicap. I suspected my cabin mates felt the same way. As a result, we had no bullies in camp. I am sure we all lacked the desire to inflict pain on anyone else. So, peace reigned in the cabin.

But quiet did not always prevail. The babies saw to that. We always had a few babies in the cabin—kids who would whimper for their mommy after "Lights Out" or who would wet the bed in the night. We would resolve these disturbances ourselves, not waiting for the night patrol to intervene. To the whimperers, someone would call out, "Aw, shut up already, and go to sleep!" As for the bed wetters, we ignored them, determined to let the counselor deal with the problem in the morning.

There was a key to nighttime success. You needed to fall asleep quickly and then sleep all the way through until "Rise and Shine." Most nights, I could do this. Sleep came easily those nights because I was tired out by all the fresh air and activity of camp life. On occasion, however, one does have to get up in the middle of the night. If you found yourself in this situation, you quickly real-ized you were facing several problems. First, you had to remember that, unlike your home, there was no bathroom down the hall. You would have to find the outhouse somewhere out there in the forest. Second, you would have to remember to put on your shoes. The outhouse was down a hill in the forest and not down a carpeted hallway. Third, you would have to decide whether you needed to wear a jacket. Summer nights in Wisconsin can get chilly. Fourth, you would have to exercise caution so as not to wake your cabin mates. They would not appreciate a slammed cabin door. With all this running through your mind, you might wonder why there weren't more incidents of bed-wetting. Finally, once outside the cabin, you had to actually find the outhouse. For a boy who is blind or partially sighted, this could be a daunting task. Alone in the forest, you would have to remember the path you trod before in the company of counselor or cabin mates. Then, taking a deep breath, you would aim yourself in what you hoped was the right direction. A boy in this predicament, however, should always remember that he has an alternative. If he cannot find the outhouse and gets really desperate, he can always pee on the ground—away from the cabin, downhill, and with the wind. I managed fairly well under these scary circumstances. Notwithstanding a few stumbles and more than a few scratches, I never lost my way on a solo nighttime adventure. On a few occasions, I even helped a boy who was totally blind successfully find his way.

\* \* \*

Finding the outhouse at night should not be how a partially sighted boy measures the value of his camp experience. Yet, these night adventures were symbolic of what was happening. I had accomplished something—on my own. True, as a Lions camper, I was rarely all on my own, strictly speaking. I always had a counselor nearby to help me find and identify my food in the dining hall, to warn me before I walked into a tree on a hike in the forest, or to prevent my drowning in the lake. But, I was on my own in an important sense. For a time, I lived beyond parents and teachers—out of touch with and out of reach of the familiar reference points of home and school. This was a new experience for me. For the first time in my life, I experienced a taste of independence. It was a brief taste, lasting for only the week at camp—a week that always passed too quickly. I enjoyed the brief taste of independence and eventually developed an appetite for more.

Also, for the first time in my life, I experienced a sense of solidarity with other vision-impaired kids. Even though I had good friends in my Sight Saving classroom at school, I never developed a "Band of Brothers" attitude toward them. We did not have an "us against them" climate in our room. I enjoyed being with my classmates; I did not want to be like them. Even though most of my classmates could see better than I, I was smarter than they. Besides, we always had the kids in the regular classroom to contend with. They could see far away things and hit a softball. At school, therefore, I always had an underlying sense of disappointment, frustration, and isolation. I was constantly reminded of what I was not—of what I was lacking. In my own mind, I was convinced, more than occasionally, that I was a loser and an outcast. At camp, however, there were no disappointments or frustrations. There were no losers or outcasts either. Everyone was in the same boat. No one was better off than anyone else; no one had an advantage that others lacked. We were all the same, and we were all there to have fun. For the first time in my life, I had an inkling of what would take many years to understand and accept. "This is what I am," my camp experience suggested. "This is who I am. It's not so bad."

\* \* \*

As with all good things, camp had to come to an end. The final day of camp was an adventure in itself. The camp commandant decided that we should not pack wet swim trunks in our suitcases for the trip home. So, he decreed that the boys could take the morning swim but only in the nude—swim trunks to be kept dry at all costs. Now, I knew nothing of sexuality; the terms "gender politics" and "women's liberation" had not been invented yet; and I knew little of the civil rights struggles of the day. I was only around 10 years old at the time. Yet, somehow, I believed the "no trunks" decree was unfair. What about the girls? Why couldn't they swim on the last day, just as they had (in separate sessions from the boys) every other day? Why couldn't the girls swim in the nude? Oh, sure, the beach was right next to the boys' cabins, but so what? We wouldn't spy on the naked girls. Even if we tried, what could we see? We were all blind or vision impaired. I did not understand this apparent case of discrimination. I did not, however, let it stop me from swimming on the last day of camp.

Skinny-dipping was fun—at least for the first two years. Something changed in the third year. That year, we had, for the first time, a female lifeguard. Now, a bunch of naked preteen boys might not mean much to a college woman, but having a female lifeguard meant something to me. I did not want to go skinny-dipping that year. I did not know why I was so reluctant. I suppose I was simply nervous about a woman seeing me naked. So, I wore my swimsuit down to the beach that day and sat on the pier next to the lifeguard. Carefully keeping my suit dry, I splashed my feet in the cool water. I told myself that, in boycotting the nude swimming, I was striking a blow for women's rights. I didn't say that to the lifeguard, though. She stood near me on the pier, watching the swimmers. She asked me why I wasn't swimming. I mumbled some excuse. I certainly could not go into the water now! I would have to undress right in front of her. I could not do that. She blew her whistle a few minutes later. Mercifully, swim period was over.

We packed our dry swim trunks (but wet towels), climbed the hill for the last time, said good-bye to counselors and staff, and boarded the bus for home—home to the familiar, the urban.

* * *

On the long trip home that third year, I considered what camp had done for me. I had made nothing (or, at least nothing I cared to bring home). I had made no lifelong friendships. I had made no contacts to help me in a career. I had won no medals. (The only competition had been the treasure hunt, and we had consumed the prize.) I had won no games. (One does not play baseball or basketball at Lions Camp.) One might say that, except for the suntan that would fade before school started in September, I had nothing tangible to show for my time in the wilderness. I had feelings, though. I felt gratitude to the Lions for giving this opportunity to kids with impaired vision. I felt appreciation for the work of the counselors—all destined, no doubt, to be fine teachers and social workers. I felt pleasure in the brief taste of independence and "sense of self" camp had afforded. I had memories, too. I shall always remember eating Fond du Lac corn on the cob, tramping around the lake, raising and lowering the flag, singing camp songs, listening to campfire stories, winning the treasure hunt, swimming in the nude (prior to the advent of the female lifeguard), searching for the outhouse alone in the forest at night, and climbing that damned hill.

Reprinted with permission from Douglas M. Karlen, karlend@ctt.com, February 15, 2006.

Having traversed a wide range of fiction and nonfiction by the blind here, we come at the end to another piece of nonfiction by an experienced, seasoned traveler. Here we see a woman whose life is fully realized and exciting, one able to travel the world confidently and enjoy every step of the way. Here is Audrey Schading's piece about her life, appropriately entitled "Joy":

## JOY

### by Audrey Schading

"You have a very rich life," a friend commented to me when I was preparing to travel to Bahrain to participate in a professional/cultural exchange program with MIUSA (Mobility International USA), an organization that orchestrates many global, innovative programs for teens and adults with disabilities.

She's right. My life is very rich, and when I think about its richness, I am ever amazed, myself!

I believe I agreed to a specific soul contract before birth, one in which I chose to live life as a blind American woman. Of course, when I'm in a completely frustrated unhappy state, I then can never quite comprehend why I accepted physical blindness as part of my life's work; however, in my very soul, I know I did, and I realize that the understanding and knowledge will become clear as this life and beyond continues to unfold.

The gift of joy within me is astounding and boundless. Its spirit resonates each day I awake. My heart sings and dances for joy, and it flows out, everywhere I am. It, along with peace, wisdom, and comfort, becomes strong within me, radiating through me during times of darkness, despair, and general discouragement. When those times come, and I feel I am the worst of the worst, and allow myself to be surrounded with all degrees of fear and negativity, I get the reassurance deep within me that God has brought me this far in my life, and He/She will always continue to be there, no matter what.

That's what really keeps me going—to know that the entire Universe is working with me at all times, even when I forget. Although I instinctively know this but have somehow forgotten, the Universe ultimately always comes through, I then marvel at its depth of comprehension, marvel that it knows exactly what I need at all times!

It comes forth for every kind of possible (or improbable) thing imaginable. This can happen when I need assistance in innumerable situations both large and small, small as in finding the location of a doctor's office or great as in the following:

In February 2003, I was preparing to travel to Tokyo (again for MIUSA) and spent the day working on two very important projects. The first was to acquire special papers from a veterinarian at JFK Airport that would enable my guide dog Duncan to travel. After completing that task, I commenced with the second, which was to replace my passport, my original having gotten lost. Although I was near the correct address, as I'd just gotten off of the appropriate subway, I couldn't quite find the location. Someone offered assistance, which I gratefully accepted. He explained that he worked for that particular department, and could show me exactly where it was. We walked together having a light conversation.

About two minutes into our walk, he asked me if I was from Buffalo, New York. I said I was. He then asked if I used to teach English as a second language there approximately 30 years ago. Again he was correct. He then told me his name, and said he'd been in one of my adult classes. He did not know my name; however, he remembered my face. I marveled about all of this, and was even more amazed later on.

When I venture to a place on my own, I request that someone help me fill out the appropriate print information. As I was accompanied for this time, my guide offered to fill out everything, which was great. Upon handing in the paperwork, I was told I needed a witness in order to get the passport. Ordinarily, I'd be prepared to argue the fact; however, I was tired, was leaving the next morning, and needed to return to work. My new/old acquaintance/angel said he'd be a witness.

When they asked him how long he knew me, he said, "Thirty years!!"

What a blessing! I was then able to get my passport and be on my way!

That evening, as I was packing, I thought with amazement that when he'd first met me, the Universe knew there'd be a future reason for him to remember my face.

Soon after returning from Tokyo, my guide dog and I were both injured and were in serious need of medical attention. As I waited for an ambulance surrounded by caring coworkers and strangers, a veterinarian emerged, and walked toward us! In her tremendous kindness, she took my dog for necessary medical care while I went to the hospital. We both healed, and the wonderful veterinarian kept in touch with me via e-mail and cell phone. After about two weeks, I could no longer locate her by phone or e-mail. Was she a vet, or an angel stepping in to help? I don't know, and I am forever grateful to her and the many others who were there for me at an exact specific place and moment! These can be "Angels Along the Way" as singer/actress/minister Della Reece said in her book bearing that same title.

I believe we are all angels, and we have forgotten that we are. We learn from our fellow angels, and we teach them, too. And not only from those who are kind to us! Angels/people who show us difficulties and problems are our teachers, too; though, when we are in our particular hell, we don't usually remember that fact.

There is joy and gratitude resonating everywhere for me, joy in knowing that from infancy I had loving parents, friends, and teachers who patiently taught me to discover my world without vision; joy in remembering the first day I could actually read Braille letters; joy from teaching that and many other subjects to adults and children; joy from communicating in several languages; joy from having been married, from having and raising two children, and from getting to know and spend time with my grandchildren; and joy from freely walking with my guide dog, cross-country skiing, attending theater, and traveling, whether visiting family or friends nearby, traveling across the country, or to the other side of the world. There's amazement, humility, joy, and gratitude in all of it! And, I'm glad I signed up!

Audrey Schading (audrey615@verizon.net) is deeply "committed to infusing the disability perspective into international development issues." MIUSA collaborates with international agencies to ensure that people with disabilities participate fully and equally at all levels of the development process: as beneficiaries, volunteers, trainers, field staff, administrators, and policy makers. Using world-renowned consultants, MIUSA provides technical assistance to governmental and nongovernmental organizations (NGOs) working toward inclusive policy and programming. MIUSA offers organization assessments, staff training, gender planning, networking lists of disability-led NGOs, and conference presentations. MIUSA is a member of InterAction, a coalition of over 160 U.S. relief, development, and refugee agencies.

Reprinted with permission from Audrey Schading.

# 5

❖❖❖

# The Spiritual Dimensions
# of Blindness

It's always been a gift with me, hearing music the way I do. I don't
know where it comes from, it's just there and I don't question it.

Miles Davis

From the very beginning of our lives, from the first time we hear the nursery rhyme "Three Blind Mice," for example, we are primed to be aware of
blindness. It is interesting that it is three blind mice, not three deaf mice
or three deaf-mute mice. The disability of blindness has a special place in
contemporary culture: whereas in the Old Testament, illness was a sign of
divine disfavor and blindness was a particular form of God's displeasure—
but in the New Testament and the Qur'an blindness is not seen as the
result of sin. The blind are not pushed away from the sacred places and
texts as they are in the Old Testament and in ancient Judaism; when Muhammad frowns at and turns away from a blind man, Allah chastises him
for that action, and He assures Muhammad that the blind are or can be
just as ritually clean as any other human being. Allah invites the blind to
worship him and to his worship. They are not outcasts, as they are in some
societies—in old, traditional Indian society, for instance. Some are excellent musicians, writers, philosophers, poets, and thinkers. In the New
Testament and the Qur'an, they are full-fledged members of society and
hence are welcomed along with all the other disabled. Jesus and Allah
both made the point that healing and accepting the blind should be part

of anyone's ministry; and the healing of blind Bartimaeus in the New Testament is significant to our study.

Blindness in the Christian scriptures has at least two meanings—that the person is physically blind on the one level, and that she or he is inwardly blind on the spiritual level. The blind that Jesus heals are manifestly totally blind on the physical level, of course, and they are—or may be—blind inwardly too because of their prejudices, preconceptions, and close-mindedness.

## BLINDNESS IN MYSTICAL POETRY

In a dark time, the eye begins to see.

Theodore Roethke

When it is dark enough, you will see the stars.

Persian proverb

### In a Dark Time, the Eye Begins to See

In the last year of his life, in 1963, anticipating death, the mystical poet Theodore Roethke, wrote, "In a dark time, the eye begins to see," the first line of one of his best poems, a poem to be published later posthumously. He said he always wrote with a "driving sincerity,—that prime virtue of any creative worker. I write only what I believe to be the absolute truth,— even if I must ruin the theme in so doing" (quoted in Ellmann and O'Clair 777). This line and poem have mystical dimensions familiar to all mystics and students of mysticism—and possibly to all blind people, too, since the concept that in darkness the inner spiritual eye begins to see is not alien to mystical practice worldwide. We began this study by focusing on Homer, the blind seer and epic poet, in chapter 2, and it is appropriate in speaking about the spiritual dimensions of blindness that we treat the way the great American poet Theodore Roethke has spoken about seeing in the darkness, as he said he did as he anticipated death; his first line of "In a Dark Time," in four stanzas of five lines each, with a rhyming couplet at the end of each stanza, begins its mystical journey into the darkness, which paradoxically is full of light for the mystic persona:

> In a dark time, the eye begins to see I meet my shadow in the deepening shade.

He might be speaking of the way one who is learning a new way of walking finds his way "in the deepening shade," at a time when his "light" is going out, since Roethke said "that the title refers to a dark night of the soul" (787). This is a time when, as Emily Dickinson put it at the end of her poem "I heard a Fly buzz—when I died,", "I could not see to see—" (587). It is a time of spiritual darkness when the seeker develops a way of moving and being in accord with his new condition and begins to open the inner eyes, learn to cope in this darkening time by developing inner sight, insight, intuition. In baroque fashion, everything is turned into its opposite here since this is a spiritual dark night of the soul. Instead of light, he is guided by dark: "Dark, dark my light, and darker my desire" (Ellmann and O'Clair 787). This rhythmical line expresses how like a photographic negative his experience of perception of light is and how all light is now dark for him, and suddenly his soul is awakened and buzzing like a fly:

> My soul, like some heat-maddened summer fly,
>     Keeps buzzing at the sill. Which I is I? (787)

He cannot understand, perceive, or fix his own identity, does not know which "I is I," or which self is himself. Paralleling this is the opening line of another of his most mystical poems, "The Waking":

> I wake to sleep, and take my waking slow.
>     I feel my fate in what I cannot fear. (787)

He only "learn[s] by going where I have to go" (782). The moving forward is intuitive progress, accomplished through a heart-knowing, not through head-knowing.

Later in "In a Dark Time," Roethke again re-creates the experience of moving forward while blind when he expresses the purpose of this progress thus:

> A man goes far to find out what he is—
>     Death of the self in a long, tearless night. (787)

His light is in fact all darkness, wholly spiritual, and so is his desire, informed as it is by this new life and awareness of darkness he is experiencing. With this new awareness, he resolves the question of "Which I is I" by answering,

> A fallen man, I climb out of my fear.
>     The mind enters itself, and God the mind.

Here the persona and reader experience a mystical union with God, "And one is One, free in the tearing wind" (787). While before the night had been "tearless," here we are in "the tearing wind," where tears matter and flow. The mind must enter the divine in itself for God to enter the mind. While this language is obscure, the meaning is that the fallen man climbs out of his fear and joins in mystical union with God in a spiritual merging. The one individual alone melts into and joins with the Oneness of the universe, and he is "free in the tearing wind." By comparison, the blind too, in tuning in to the universal light, can use it and learn to walk and see in the darkness.

## SEEING WITH THE EYE OF THE HEART

St. Theresa and others have said that human beings are God's hands and feet and eyes and ears on earth. In Sufi mystical tradition, the divine is envisioned as dwelling within each human being, and seeing with the eye of the heart is each human being's goal. In *The Music of the Soul*, Shaykh Muhammad Sa'id al-Jamal ar-Rifa'i as-Shadhuli declares that the ideal state is one in which one is communing with God, face to face (17). He continues, "This is who you are. You see that your eye is really the eye of God. There is only one eye." The true mystic sees through God's eye. The human eye expresses human consciousness, and it is the vehicle of most silent communication between two people. The eye has been called the window of the soul, yet, according to Sufi tradition, in the next world, initially at least, all are blind. In mystical poetry the eye symbolizes poetic vision. In all mystical traditions, the mystic's ability to "read" and "write" the divine earns him or her the right to be called a mystic.

## SUFISM

Shaykh Muhammad Sa'id al-Jamal ar-Rifa'i as-Shadhuli explains, "When [a] person knows himself well, he becomes the picture of God. He sees with the eyes of God and hears with the ears of God....[God] puts the secret in every appearance...of existence. It is through existence that God sees Himself manifested" (17). Clarifying how one reaches this state of mystical communion with God and what happens when one is there, the Shaykh writes,

> When you reach the way, you search and you know who you are. Look what you...Can see then. You see your eye, and that eye is re- ally the eye of God. You are the eye of God. It is a gift from God, the

kindness of God that makes you one of His eyes, one eye. This is the way of the person who forgets all things and returns to the truth in the beginning, a child in the presence of God.

When he [or she] says, "*Allahu Akbar,*" at the moment, he is the eye of God, and the Truth of this is that at the time, all that is in this earth, this life, is finished for him. He has become absent from his soul and his mind. He meets his Love to the end which has no end. They are together and they are one thing only, without borders, without up, without down, without right or left. That is the garden to him. (17)

Later, addressing the believers, he says, "I think you [are]…the sons of God, the eyes of the truth of Muhammad" (33). He is obviously not speaking here of physical eyes, but the eyes of divine truth. Eyes like these virtually anyone can develop—the sighted or the unsighted—since they are the eyes of inner spiritual vision. He asserts, "You see your eye, and that your eye is really the eye of God." This may be difficult for many to accept or understand since we are not accustomed to hearing that our eyes are those of God. Having said that, the meaning of the line may be construed more humbly and simply if it is interpreted to mean that each person has the capacity to see with the eyes of the divine or of God as he or she understands God. Each must only be open to the divine and have a capacity for wonder and keen insight, and be open to perceiving and experiencing joy and the inner light, as Jesus said that one must become as innocent and humble as a little child in order to enter the kingdom of Heaven.

\* \* \*

The Sufi poet Rumi wrote a dialogue between a mule and a camel, a fable, about differences in sight. In the story the mule wonders why he frequently falls as he moves along the road on his way to the marketplace or falls when going down a mountainside yet, he notes, the camel never falls. He asks, "Why is that? Is it because you're destined always to be happy?" (Rumi 125). A bit self-pitying, the mule asks the camel if he is like the simple man who is beaten. Is he like

"that man of luckless nature [beaten] for breaking his vows of prayer.…
Is this me?" asked the mule. "Is this me?" (Rumi *Illustrated* 125)

Clearly the mule saw the camel as the "true believer," but the camel replies that the differences between them are brought on by the camel's higher perspective—the fact that his eyes are so much higher than the mule's:

Though every joy comes from God, there are many differences between us. I have a higher head, and therefore my eyes are higher too.
Lofty vision is a protection against injury. From the top of the mountain I can see the pathways more easily, every hollow and level, step
by step.

Then he continues, "The eye is the guide to the foot and the hand, /
For it sees...the wrong place to step." And the camel concludes, "If the
eye be pure, so the nature is pure," and "my eye is so, a child of God, not
perdition" (125).

There are various ways of seeing—physical sight is not the same as
spiritual sight, however, and here the mule acknowledges not just the
camel's higher perspective when he asks to come into his service but his
spiritual vision as well. And the latter is the source of his superiority. Here
the camel symbolizes God or Allah, while the mule represents the human
being, who comprehends the greatness of God and begs to serve Him. To
Him, human sight is much less important than spiritual insight since in
Sufism, for instance, Muhammad himself is "the Ocean of the Light,...He
[Muhammad] is the one who had the enjoyment of seeing You, the Eye of
the eyes of the Creation, the one who has been lit from the Light of Your
[God's] Brightness" (*Ocean of the Mercy* 55). In every world religion, the
divine sight is superior to human sight, physical sight. And only knowing
God matters: human beings are created for this purpose—to know God,
"Who is 'nearer to us than our jugular vein' [Q 50:16]...and Who has cre-
ated us for that possibility alone" (55).

## LOOKING WITH THE EYE OF THE HEART

Sufi masters encourage the followers of the Sufi path to follow what they
call "the straight way," walking on a straight path to God, not looking to
the left or to the right but looking directly ahead and focusing the eye
of the heart on God. Correspondingly, Jesus said to his followers, "You
are the light of the world" (Matthew 5:14). Jesus also said, "The light of
the body is the eye: if therefore thine eye be single, thy whole body will
be full of light" (Matthew 6:22), emphasizing each human being's ability
to see with the "single" eye spiritually, to see with divine eyes and insight.
In Zen Buddhism the idea of seeing with a single eye is also central to
Buddhist teachings. In the commentary, the author of *The Gateless Gate*,
says "To understand clearly one has to have just one eye" (Yamada). The
author of *Music of the Soul* expresses a similar thought when he declares,

"You are the light in this world, this weeping, sad world" (33). And everywhere in mystical literature, around the world, the light represents God. He calls it a sad world since he experiences the suffering of the world very deeply and strives constantly to alleviate that suffering. He believes that is our purpose as human beings—to help relieve the suffering of others in any way we can.

Likewise, in the mystical and literary traditions spiritual blindness is likened to and equated with spiritual, emotional, and psychological limitations or evil. Spiritual sight is the holy ability to perceive and see the deeper truth, and this has nothing to do with having real physical sight or not. We process much more information through our eyes than we do through our other senses; mystical traditions all direct would-be mystics not to use their eyes but instead to close them and listen for God's voice inside. They develop an inner knowing and inner sight called "seeing with the eyes of the heart." The mystic must work conscientiously through prayer and meditation toward a condition of being blind to this world so as to hear and see and sense the divine inside himself—to see with the eye of the heart and experience the divine dwelling within. Shaykh Muhammad Sa'id al-Jamal ar-Rifa'i as-Shadhuli says that once a believer discovers God inside himself or herself he or she is enraptured, and "you weep because you see that you lost so much time when you lived in the world outside, 'Why did I live like a blind person in the world?' You weep because you begin to see through clean eyes when you walk in this station" (*Music* 50). The blind are to the normally sighted as the sighted are to those who see through the eye of the heart. In his book *The Stories of the Prophets*, the Shaykh says of this way of seeing,

> A blind person has eyes, but he cannot see because He [God] did not send the quality of seeing through his eyes. But when He give you the seeing, you see with the Eye of Allah, with the quality of Allah. The outside eye is like a shadow, but behind that is the seeing eye. (141)

Seeing with God's sight is infinitely better than seeing through human eyes.

In *The Music of the Soul*, he writes about how seeing can actually imperil the souls of the sighted. When Joseph of the Old Testament in the Bible and in the Torah appeared in Egypt, he was so handsome, according to Sufi lore, that women became distracted and enraptured by his beauty.

In a transport of rapture, some cut themselves and felt no pain, believing he was a angel:

> They exclaim, "Is this a human being?" (Qur'an 12:31). In *The Music of the Soul*, the Shaykh says of Joseph's transformative effect on those who saw him:

> [Joseph] was a human being, but their eyes saw a noble angel. They saw his inside image in which he was an angel, and in that moment they did not see his outside [image] which was that of a human being. Therefore it is said:
> *And what is it, but that I see it suddenly*
> *And I am dazzled by it, knowing yet not knowing.* (Music of the Soul 431)

The sight of Joseph, his dazzling angelic appearance, overwhelmed the local women. Although Joseph was both a human being and a prophet, his beauty was so overpowering that they considered him an angel, and hence in their excitement and ecstasy the women cut their hands without feeling the cuts. Their eyes were opened to his divine reality, which they believed to be angelic and may have been. This reality is a realm open to any human being whose inner eyes are opened.

Yet in his book *The Stories of the Prophets,* the Shayhk says that Joseph "is not a human being like they thought, but an angel different from any human being." He was "the complete light" (*Stories of the Prophets* 127). So his actual being encompasses the qualities of human being, angel and prophet. This example illustrates how something seen can disrupt the lives of those who see what they can't understand. Similarly these women were astounded at Joseph's appearance and his being, imagining him to be an angel, some supernatural being: spiritual shock occurs "when such unveilings come in an unfamiliar way without being recognized by the self" (*Music of the Soul* 431). If a person is born blind, he or she can experience a similar occurrence if sight is restored suddenly: "Such is the case of a person who is born blind and is suddenly able to see and know the things around him" (431). People born blind can sometimes be too overwhelmed to understand what is happening to them, and they can panic if sight is restored too suddenly. They become bewildered by the onrush of unfamiliar visual sense impressions and can actually be incapable of seeing because they cannot deal with this unfamiliar onslaught on the visual cortex. This story has been told in the film *At First Sight*, in which the blind main character, played by Val Kilmer, has seen nothing for many years and is suddenly able to see. He panics because his brain cannot apprehend what is happening. The man is not able to cope with the overload of sensory input and begins screaming, sending everyone away, quite psychologically distressed that he has not been able to use his new gift of sight. He has to be retrained in seeing since it is a skill each sighted person uses unconsciously, while the blind who recover their sight have to learn how to link sight and cognition in order to understand what they are seeing.

## SECOND SIGHT

Often the blind are credited with or understood to possess enhanced perception of the truth, or second sight, since they can pick up on nonvisual clues and insights into another person's character while the sighted may rely too heavily on their powers of sight to bring them all necessary information. Many blind people claim that their senses are far more acute than those of the sighted and feel a certain modest superiority over sighted people in this one area. Our culture tends to think that seeing is believing, while the blind develop their own, alternative ways of knowing. For the blind person to move into mysticism may be much easier since he or she is never distracted by information coming in from the visual cortex. That is not to say that one has to be blind to have mystical knowledge, however.

In the Sufi tradition, Sufis on the path to God frequently have gatherings called *Hawwahs* where they chant certain verses and prayers over and over again. Then, having purified themselves in the process, they visualize the name of God, first, for an hour staring at it with eyes wide open. Next, they seek to bring the name of God into inner sight by visualizing it with their eyes closed. Both the sighted and the unsighted must do this for two hours or more at some religious gatherings so as to bring reality of God inside themselves and make God part of inner vision, part of each person.

The sign asking everyone to "Visualize world peace"—humorously parodied by some as "Visualize whirled peas"—used to be a common bumper sticker frequently plastered on cars; and it's commonly thought that the ability to visualize any event or transformation can help bring it about in ways we don't yet understand. By extension, the Sufi custom of prayer and visualizing the name of God is a clear attempt to bring the divine inside and to internalize God. The Prophet Mohammad said, "My solace is in prayer, the cooling of the eyes" (*Ocean of the Mercy* 134). It is a practical approach to mysticism, and Sufism is said to provide the most direct path to enlightenment, or the mystical union with God.

In sum, if spiritual and subtle human communication are linked with inner sight, spiritual insight comes from inner vision, which might actually be enhanced when one becomes blind. This may be a positive and unexpected dimension of blindness. Since on the physical plane, the blind who strive hard to master independent activity eventually develop facial vision, or echo location, so on the spiritual plane they come to connect more easily with the divine, their higher power, or with God, because they are not distracted by visual cues and the superficial appearance of each person or object but are able to focus on and use all their other senses to apprehend a person, an object, or a situation or environment. Many nurses, doctors, ophthalmologists, and other professionals who work with the blind over the course of their lifetime believe the blind see with the eye of their heart. In some sense, they are more inwardly inclined to be oriented toward mysticism; they take more naturally to mysticism. If the mystic happens to be a blind person or the blind person a mystic, the light is internal; he or she experiences the divine within himself or herself. If the person sees spiritually in the darkness, blindness could be seen as a great gift, as John Hull claimed it was. It can truly be a way to advance confidently on a spiritual path toward the divine—toward God.

## THE CHRISTIAN OLD TESTAMENT PERSPECTIVE ON BLINDNESS

Certainly ancient humans, in intellectual blindness, considered physical blindness either a curse of God or a retribution for wrongdoing. God was seen as the creator of blindness: "And they smote the men that were at the door of the house with blindness, both small and great: so that they wearied themselves to find the door" (Gen. 19:11). In Exodus 23, one is rewarded with blindness for siding with the unjust against the just: "And thou shalt take no gift: for the gift blindeth the wise, and perverteth the words of the righteous" (Exod. 23:8). If one receives a reward—blood money—for a false testimony against the righteous, "the gift"—money or other reward—blinds the wise, either physically or mentally and spiritually. Blindness is specifically the retribution for accepting a bribe: "Behold, here I am: witness against me before the LORD, and before his anointed: whose ox have I taken? or whose ass have I taken? or whom have I defrauded? whom have I oppressed? or of whose hand have I received any bribe to blind mine eyes therewith?" (1 Sam. 12:3).

The unregenerate David, sadly, hated the blind it is said: "And the king and his men went to Jerusalem unto the Jebusites, the inhabitants of the land: which spake unto David, saying, Except thou take away the blind and the lame, thou shalt not come in hither: thinking, David cannot come in hither" (2 Sam. 5:6). Later on, Elisha prays that God might smite his enemies with blindness: "And when they came down to him, Elisha prayed unto the LORD, and said, Smite this people, I pray thee, with blindness. And he smote them with blindness according to the word of Elisha" (2 Kings 6:18). Zephaniah speaks of striking those who have sinned with blindness (1:17). And in order to prevent the success of evil men in war, Zachariah warns, "In that day, saith the LORD, I will smite every horse with astonishment, and his rider with madness: and I will open mine eyes upon the house of Judah, and will smite every horse of the people with blindness" (12:4). Without horses that could see, it was impossible for the army to triumph.

Of course, it is against divine law to put obstacles in the way of the blind: "Thou shalt not curse the deaf, nor put a stumbling block before the blind but shalt fear thy God: I am the LORD" (Lev. 19:14). And further, those who interfere with the blind will be cursed: "Cursed be he that maketh the blind to wander out of the way. And all the people shall say, Amen." (Deut. 18:27)

Correspondingly, it is blessed to help the blind: Job asserts in one of his speeches, "I was eyes to the blind, and feet was I to the lame" (29:15).

More hopefully, Isaiah recounts, "Then the eyes of the blind shall be opened, and the ears of the deaf shall be unstopped" (35:5). And the prophet's mission is to help illuminate the blind: "To open the blind eyes, to bring out the prisoners from the prison, and them that sit in darkness out of the prison house" (42:7). The divine mission is to open everyone's eyes so that they may see with spiritual sight and insight—to see divine reality.

Unfortunately, in Judaism and in the earliest times, the blind were not allowed to approach the Holy of Holies: "For whatsoever man he be that hath a blemish, he shall not approach: a blind man, or a lame, or he that hath a flat nose, or any thing superfluous (Lev. 21:18). No such person could be a rabbi or priest. Thankfully this prejudice, born of the fear that the blind were blind because of some sin, has not continued into modern times. Similar to this is a line slightly further on in the Pentateuch: "Blind, or broken, or maimed, or having a wen, or scurvy, or scabbed, ye shall not offer these unto the LORD, nor make an offering by fire of them upon the altar unto the LORD" (Lev. 22:22). Elsewhere, in Deuteronomy, the instruction is given not to sacrifice blind animals to the Lord: "And if there be any blemish therein, as if it be lame, or blind, or have any ill blemish, thou shalt not sacrifice it unto the LORD thy God" (15:21). Isaiah proclaims, "And I will bring the blind by a way that they knew not; I will lead them in paths that they have not known: I will make darkness light before them, and crooked things straight. These things will I do unto them, and not forsake them" (Isaiah 42:16). This is one of the most beautiful promises that the prophet makes, and he follows it by encouraging and commanding the blind to look (inwardly presumably), to examine themselves: "Hear, ye deaf; and look, ye blind, that ye may see" (Isaiah 42:18). Hence any blind person who examines himself or herself, who meditates and goes within to align with God, is following this biblical command.

Some Jewish men arise in the morning and give thanks they were not born a woman since women were, due to their domestic responsibilities and for other reasons, excluded from many of acts of worship and religious services Jewish men participated in. No one today would give thanks aloud for not being born blind or deaf or lame, but in the Qur'an and in the Bible, verses indicate that the blind, lame, and deaf—anyone who wasn't considered normal—were not allowed to approach the divine or enter into the presence in the Holy of Holies.

## JESUS'S HEALING MIRACLES—HEALING BLINDNESS

In the Bible, there are many instances of Jesus healing the blind; at least one blind man thanks him for this divine act of mercy. Here the blind are seen as victims. Like the poor, they are helpless until the Son of man comes along to heal them. In the Qur'an, Allah says that He could blind men or make them deaf as a punishment for sins committed, and there is some indication in the Bible that blindness is the reward of sinfulness—or perhaps the sins of the fathers, ancestral sin. Still, Jesus heals the blind, in a sense forgiving them and releasing them into new life. Blindness in the Judeo-Christian Bible, then, indicates a condition of disease that divine intervention can heal and dispel. The blind can be freed from their former condition, an existence absent from God, and brought into seeing the divine truth: in a reversal of the ancient myth, eyes healed, they at last see the reality of the one true God. They join the community of believers.

Throughout the New Testament, Jesus heals a variety of physical impairments and illnesses, like leprosy; he even raises Lazarus, a sick girl who died, and arguably others from the dead. The majority of his miracles are healing miracles, and in due course, he also heals blindness effectively and often since the blind frequently followed him, along with the lame and the sick, pleading with him to heal them. The first mention of this phenomenon is in the Book of Matthew: "And when Jesus departed thence, two blind men followed him, crying, and saying, Thou son of David, have mercy on us" (9:27). First he tested the blind men's faith by inquiring, "Do you believe that I am able to do this?" (9:28), and when they answered, "Yes, Lord," he touched their eyes and replied, "According to your faith will it be done unto you, and their sight was restored" (29). He sternly enjoined them not to speak of their healing with anyone. Later in Matthew, echoing Isaiah, Jesus spoke of a time when "the blind receive their sight, and the lame walk, the lepers are cleansed, and the deaf hear, the dead are raised up, and the poor have the gospel preached to them" (11:5). He is describing his own ministry on earth.

The blind in the New Testament are often characterized as demanding, and understandably so: "Then was brought unto him one possessed with a devil, blind, and dumb: and he healed him, insomuch that the blind and dumb both spake and saw" (Matthew 12:22). As his ministry grew and his miracles became better known, anyone who was physically challenged or impaired or ill came to him: "Great multitudes came unto him, having with them those that were lame, blind, dumb, maimed, and many others, and cast them down at Jesus' feet; and he healed them" (Matthew 15:30).

The writer of the Gospel of Mark treats these healings of the blind with greater detail, and the blind he describes seem more helpless and gentle, less demanding. In the book of Mark, just before Jesus's triumphal entry into Jerusalem, Jesus heals one blind man who's given a name and a lineage: blind Bartimaeus. "And they came to Jericho: and as he went out of Jericho with his disciples and a great number of people, blind Bartimaeus, the son of Timaeus, sat by the highway side begging" (19:46). His story comes to life, as Bartimaeus himself does, when he realizes Jesus is near: "When he heard that it was Jesus of Nazareth, he began to shout, 'Jesus, Son of David, have mercy on me!'" (47). Those around him tried to silence and scold him, but he went on shouting. "And Jesus stood still, and commanded him to be called. And they call the blind man, saying unto him, 'Be of good comfort, rise; he calleth thee'" (49). He asks Bartimaeus what he wants, and he replies, "Rabbi, I want to see" (51). And Jesus answers, "Go . . . your faith has healed you" (52). His faith in God has healed him and made him whole.

There is another version of the healing of a man born blind in the Gospel of John, which contains comparatively fewer accounts of healing miracles but which goes into far greater depth about the healing of a man born blind in John 9:1–41. Jesus puts a paste or "clay" made of mud and saliva on this man's eyes (John 9:6), and then he tells him to "'Go . . . wash in the Pool of Siloam' (this word means Sent)." And he does and returns "seeing" (7–8). Others are astounded that he now can see, and some even say that it is not the same man; but he replies, "I am the man" (9). And the day he'd been healed was a Sabbath, so the Pharisees said, 'This man is not from God, for he does not keep the Sabbath.' But others asked, "'How could a sinner do such miraculous signs?'" (16). And "the Jews still did not believe that he had been blind and had received his sight until they sent for the man's parents." But they merely said that they did not know how the man had received his sight and that he was an adult, so he should be asked. The Book of John then records that they said this only because they knew the Jews had declared that "anyone who acknowledged that Jesus was the Christ would be put out of the synagogue" (22). When he himself was asked, the healed man stood up bravely for Jesus and his healing, answering them, "I have told you already, and you did not listen. Why do you want to hear it again? Do you want to become his disciples, too?" (27). Hence he challenges them, adopts an attitude of defiance, so they "hurled insults at him and said, 'You are this fellow's disciple! We are disciples of Moses! We know that God spoke to Moses, but as for this fellow, we don't even know where he comes from'" (28–29). And the man replied, "'Now that is remarkable! You don't know where he comes from, yet he opened my eyes. We know that God does not listen to sinners. He listens to the godly man who does his will. Nobody ever heard of opening the eyes of a man born blind. If this man were not from God, he could do nothing" (30–32). Certainly the inquisitors wanted to maintain that Jesus was a mere human being. They were under the illusion that only Moses and the prophets of old could speak with God or heal. Yet the man born blind stood up to them, asserting that Jesus was someone to whom God listened, someone who had opened and healed his eyes; therefore he had to be a holy man. Muhammad was persecuted for many years in similar ways: others attacked him for setting himself up as a superior, godly man, one to whose prayers God listened, one under God's special protection. Muhammad met similar fierce opposition, and he had to fight warring tribes and many groups of people who for their own reasons desired to maintain the status quo and who believed they needed to repulse him and deny the truth of his mission of divine outpouring.

The Gospel of John describes one last element in the story of this man who'd been healed of blindness: those who called him in to cross-examine him about his healing threw him out (34). So when Jesus heard about this, he found him and asked him, "'Do you believe in the Son of Man?' 'Who is he, sir?' [Bartimaeus] asked. 'Tell me so that I may believe in him.' Jesus said, 'You have now seen him; in fact, he is the one speaking with you.' Then the man said, 'Lord, I believe,' and he worshiped him" (35–38). On one level the incident illustrates the way Jesus increased his cohort of believers through individual acts of healing (although he always tried to keep as many healings as possible secret); yet on another level this event provokes a showdown with the Pharisees who are onto him: they heard him reply to the man he'd healed, "For judgment I have come into this world, so that the blind will see and those who see will become blind" (39)—clearly a statement he means both literally and metaphorically in the second part. Yet they took this general, all-encompassing statement literally and asked if he intended to imply they were blind (40). But he answered, "If you were blind, you would not be guilty of sin; but now that you claim you can see, your guilt remains." He shows here that of course blindness is not simply determined by inability to see and unwillingness to see God in the person of Jesus Christ; it is also a matter of the orientation and openness of one's heart and spirit. He may have chosen to heal those born blind in part because the transformation they experienced was more dramatic and immediate than, say, the transformation of the healing of those born deaf or mute. Always those who are healed are those who believe and who are more open-minded and open-hearted, less set in their ways than these particular Pharisees, whose goal seems to be entrapment.

In an exegetical class presentation of John 9:1–41 on May 1, 2008, at Church Divinity School of the Pacific, Judy Lebens said this about "The Theology of the Text (Lebens Handout in BS 1010)":

> The presence of this particular blind man was an occasion in which need evoked the miracle. Giving sight to the blind enabled Jesus to lay claim to his identity as 'the light of the world'. The need in this miracle was for God's works to be made manifest in a setting which was steeped in Mosaic Law.
>
> Jesus chose to heal on the Sabbath to demonstrate that the restrictions attached to Sabbath law were designed by men and not by God. Rather than a compassionate act, Jesus' healing of the man born blind was to introduce Jewish society [to] the kingdom of God in the person of his son, the Christ. In healing the blind man, Jesus brings him from the darkness into light in an effort to demonstrate the infinite possibilities of life in the light.
>
> In these stories, Jesus proves who he is, he diagnoses humanity's problems in the spiritual blindness of the Jews, and he very clearly describes what is necessary for conversion. However, he broke Sabbath law, therefore damaging his credibility in the eyes of the Pharisees who labeled him a sinner. (5)

Obviously much is at play in this story. It's a crucial step on Jesus's path of ministry, part of his unfolding of the divine plan, part of his justification for claiming he is 'the light of the world. I would disagree with Lebens in that I see it also as an act of compassion while at the same time he is introducing society to "the kingdom of God" by demonstrating his divinely endowed powers of healing. While for the theologian, of course, the latter goal may be more important, for those coping with the onset of blindness the compassionate healing itself and the role of faith and belief in bringing it about are more important.

In the section entitled "Food For Thought," at the end of her exegetical presentation, Judy Lebens asks, "Was healing this man in the man's best interest or was he simply used as a conduit to introduce God's living, breathing salvific presence in the world?" Citing the passage from Leviticus quoted above that commands, "Do not...put a stumbling block in front of the blind, but fear your God....Do not do anything that endangers your neighbor's life," Lebens reasons,

> According to God's covenant with the Jews, the blind were to be protected. So, what are the implications for this man who, although he spent his life as a beggar, was protected by society? Now that he could see, was he in physical danger? Would he still have a place to live? Would he continue to beg for alms or would he be thrown outside the city walls?

These are profound, probing questions that engage our thoughts and sympathy: one certainly hopes he would still have a place to live since the city's compassion ought to extend to those who've been blind for a lifetime and then are miraculously healed. Some accommodation should be made for someone who may not yet have a trade or means to support himself in the absence of public assistance, a formal welfare system as we know it or a government-funded allowance for disability. One hopes that Jesus made some arrangements for the formerly blind man, and it's heartening to note that presumably he also had his parents to fall back on in a pinch. It seems extreme to assert that he might now be in physical danger or that he might be thrown outside the city walls, especially as he has done nothing wrong, has broken no law. Certainly Jesus healed him and changed his life out of love for him, so he would not have let him be cast aside or ostracized afterward.

He did this to emphasize the spiritual blindness of those in contemporary society. We have a cultural concept of spiritual blindness, whereas we do not have a conception of spiritual deafness or spiritual muteness, so Jesus focuses specifically on the blind to advance his divine mission on earth and prove his healing powers as the Son of man.

Ironically, although Luke says he is a physician, his Gospel contains fewer precise descriptions of such miracles but instead quotes the passage from Isaiah assuring the faithful that when the Messiah comes, the blind will be healed and the lame will walk, "The Spirit of the Lord is upon me, because he hath anointed me to preach the gospel to the poor; he hath sent me to heal the brokenhearted, to preach deliverance to the captives, and recovering of sight to the blind, to set at liberty them that are bruised" (14:8). He repeats Jesus's injunction to invite the blind, the poor, the maimed and lame to any feast, as they are the more deserving and more grateful: "But when thou makest a feast, call the poor, the maimed, the lame, the blind" (14:13). In the parable of the great banquet, he tells of a lord of a great house who gives an order to a servant that seems to run counter to common practice or local customs: "So that servant came, and shewed his lord these things. Then the master of the house being angry said to his servant, Go out quickly into the streets and lanes of the city, and bring in hither the poor, and the maimed, and the halt, and the blind" (14:21). Angered that those he invited are not wearing the correct garments, the lord orders his servants to scour the bushes and streets, the roads and country lanes, to find those who are willing to come celebrate and eat his banquet with him. This implies that blind are more ready to listen and more open to receive divine truth, the divine message, than others are—others who are engaged in business and the ordinary work of life. This injunction sounds almost like a punishment for those who are too caught up in trivia to realize when someone important arrives or issues an invitation or when something momentous is occurring: "I tell you," the master tells his servant in the parable, "not one of those men who were invited will get a taste of my banquet" (Luke 14:25). This parable invites many interpretations, but essentially its message is that many are called, the blind among them, and often it is those whom society considers the least successful or useful who hear the call of the divine.

The Gospels of Luke and John continue in the same vein, occasionally associating blindness with the prophesies of Isaiah and the Second Coming and at other times referring to the phenomenon of the blind leading the blind Luke observes in his contemporary society. "And he spake a parable unto them, Can the blind lead the blind? shall they not both fall into the ditch?" (Luke 39:6). The nation was spiritually blind at this juncture and Jesus knows he has come to open the eyes of these blind citizens, although he realizes that the longer his ministry is kept secret, the longer he can remain alive. This abstract negative perception of blindness runs through these biblical books and through the Qur'an because each prophet comes to the earth to heal and help—both literally and figuratively prophets seek to enable the blind to see. The tension between spiritual and physical blindness runs through all the healing miracles, emphasizing Jesus's purpose, which is salvation.

## BLINDNESS IN THE QUR'AN AND IN MEISTER ECKHART

In the Qur'an, at the beginning of the chapter "Suratu Abasa" ("He Frowned") is the following passage: "He frowned and turned away— because the blind man came to him. / And yet for all you knew he might have been purified— / or reminded [of the Truth] and then have profited by the reminder" (80:1–3). This is a warning not to turn away from the blind because they too can be purified and may be.

Muhammad had been speaking to another man, who he'd been trying to convert despite that man's indifference. Then a blind man with genuine questions about the faith approaches Muhammad, and he frowns at the blind man and turns away. This displeased Allah, who punished him as a result of his rudeness to the blind man and because he'd ignored a man of sincere desire to know Allah in favor of a man who was more prestigious and wealthy. Muhammad had been misled, dazzled by the first man's better looks and higher standing in the community. After his punishment for this mistake, Muhammad learned to look deep into the heart of any person who approached him and see his or her true worth, seeing spiritually rather than with his physical eyes.

One important hadith, or a confirmed official saying of Muhammad, dwells on sight and blindness and holds warm assurance and hope for the blind or near-blind: "The beloved Messenger... once revealed these words directly from Allah.... Whenever I deprive my servants of their two eyes in this earthly world, they receive from Me nothing less than eyes that can already see Paradise" ("Hadith 34," *101 Diamonds* 77). This rich, heart-warming promise should inspire anyone facing blindness or loss of vision. The blind have eyes "that can already see Paradise"—if one knows how to look! Correspondingly, Meister Eckhart wrote, "The eye with which I see God is the same eye as that with which He sees me. My eye and the eye of God are one eye, one vision, one knowledge, and one love" (270). May we all learn how to look and see Paradise within.

## SPIRITUAL PRACTICES FOR THE BLIND

All of the major world religions have guidelines and practices for meditation and contemplation that are primarily aimed at sighted people. In many cases, for instance, while meditating or contemplating, practitioners are usually advised to close their eyes so as to better focus and still the mind. Depending on the faith tradition or practice, the goal is either to gain a closer relationship with God or to come to a realization as to who one really is. Alternatively, such practices can be valuable just to gain a more peaceful and relaxed state of mind—to deal with tensions brought on by everyday life whether or not as part of a spiritual journey. Indeed, many who describe themselves as atheists and not as followers of any world tradition still meditate just for the clear benefits they gain from daily meditation.

Formal guidelines and practices specifically for the blind seem rare, but intuitively they follow from those given to sighted people so we can attempt to present some here on that basis. First, though, a word about terminology. As is all too often the case, different people use the same word in quite different ways. In the case of the terms *meditation* and *contemplation* while it is a little overly simplistic to say so, in general these terms mean the opposite in Western teachings compared to Eastern teachings. Within the Christian tradition, for instance, to "meditate" usually means to sit calmly with eyes open and take a phrase or perhaps a passage from the Bible, and reflect upon the words. To "contemplate," by contrast, usually means to sit in silence, often with eyes closed, and try to just be still and silent most often by focusing on a single word that is repeated over and over again. This method is also called "centering prayer" in many traditions. In Eastern traditions, however, to "meditate" covers a range of practices that usually involve either sitting quietly in complete silence (the extreme example being *zazen*) or repeating a phrase or word over and over again in one's head.

Treating, first, Christian meditation, clearly any of these practices can be done by the blind by simply substituting the reading of a phrase or passage with reading in Braille or listening to a recording of the words. In its simplest form, you would read the phrase or passage in Braille, or listen to it, and then sit in silence for, say, five minutes trying not to intellectualize about the words but just let them "speak" to you in the silence. Then you might repeat this one or more times. And of course this can be done alone or in a small group. With a small group you may want to have a brief discussion afterward, or you may decide to skip any discussion because it may disturb the feeling of peace you have gained by the meditation session.

As to Christian-style "contemplation" or "centering prayer," here is where you may wish to experiment with what works best for you. The goal is to still the mind and become centered on God, which for most sighted people is best achieved by closing their eyes so that they are not distracted by what they see. Just as sighted practitioners will often set an alarm to go off after, say, 5 or 10 minutes of contemplation, you may wish to set an alarm to go off to let you know when 5 or 10 minutes have passed. A simple example of this practice would be for you to chose a simple word or very short phrase—perhaps from the Bible if that is your tradition—and aim to repeat it over and over again to yourself in silence for a brief period. Take a break and then perhaps try a session again. As you grow in your practice you may take longer periods, but just 5 minutes a day can often result in substantial reduction in stress levels and make you much more peaceful.

This technique works, too, for Middle Eastern practices like Sufi meditation, or "remembrance," which often involves the repetition of a word or short phrase, sometimes silently in one's mind, sometimes out loud. Clearly, using earplugs or headphones to reduce sound while you meditate or contemplate will make most sense when you are doing silent repetitions. Similarly for Eastern meditation practices that also call for the repetition of a word or short phrase, do it either silently to yourself or out loud. Or you may wish to just listen to repetitive sounds through headphones, such as gently chiming bells or a soundtrack of monks chanting.

One exception when it comes to Eastern meditation techniques is *zazen* from the Zen Buddhist tradition. Here the goal of sitting zazen is to still the mind and just be in the moment; fully mindful and attentive to everything that is going on in the present moment. The goal is to still the endless chatter that goes on in most of us when we try to just sit and be quiet. Guidelines for sighted people sitting zazen usually instruct them to not entirely close their eyes, and indeed many sighted people practice zazen with their eyes wide open in contrast to closed-eye Eastern meditation practices. By all means experiment with reducing sound around you, too, since you may be pleasantly surprised by the results, which may be similar to those gained by sighted people who sit zazen with their eyes closed. That said, many blind practitioners of zazen report that they find it best to practice no differently from sighted people sitting with their eyes closed.

Sitting zazen is easy to describe but hard to practice for many people. In essence, all one is doing is sitting still for a period of time—5 to 10 minutes at first—seeking to still your mind and just be present in the moment. This may sound simple, but for most of us it is harder than you might first think. As you sit in silence you will probably find your mind racing with commentary and chatter in your head ("Did I turn off the iron?" "What shall we have for dinner tonight?" "I wonder if I was too harsh when speaking to Suzy earlier today"). Formal zazen involves sitting on a cushion with your legs crossed in what is called a full-lotus position, back straight, and with your hands in a formal position, one palm lying on top of the other face up and with your thumbs lightly touching. But sitting comfortably, even if for you that is on a straight-backed chair rather than sitting on the floor, is key. Traditionally, sighted persons sit with eyes partly open, looking down at roughly a 45-degree angle and often facing a wall to minimize what they are seeing. The reason this is done, especially for those starting zazen, is to lessen the chance that practitioners fall asleep or go too much into their head. Clearly, the bind or visually impaired person will need to focus on breathing at first to try to avoid getting lost in thought or feeling too tired. Breathing deeply as low down in your body as you can (so-called belly breathing) and counting your breaths is advisable at first. Then you can move on to focusing on your breath without counting, and from there eventually to not paying attention to your breathing at all—just being in the moment, let everything just be as it is.

If you are interested in pursuing one or more of these forms of meditation or contemplation then we would encourage you to explore any of the numerous books on the subjects, many of which are available in talking books or Braille.

In summary, whether or not you are following a spiritual path or faith tradition, meditation and contemplation can be excellent ways to reduce stress and become calmer.

# 6

## Current Insights into Visual Impairment and Vision Loss or Change

Making the blind see was once called a miracle. As we have expanded our understanding of evolution, genetics, and nanotechnology, chances are that "miraculous" cures will become as commonplace as those claimed by faith-healers past and present.

Gerald Weissmann, MD, editor in chief of the *FASEB Journal*

As we have seen in previous chapters, the blind are not handicapped or lesser people than sighted people but are often as capable if not more capable than they. Yet despite this, society still tends to look down upon those they misguidedly think of as having handicaps. Certainly, we are more enlightened in Western culture than we once were, but we have some way to go before we cease marginalizing those who are different from ourselves.

### WHAT THE FUTURE HOLDS

A decade into the 21st century we are discovering that the simplistic ideas we had of the future were fundamentally flawed. We saw a future of flying cars and colonies on the moon and Mars, and humankind heading for

nearby star systems by 2010. Somewhere in this view of the future we anticipated a time when technology would evolve to a point that sight could
be given back to those who had lost it. Well, in the last five years or so science has indeed reached the point where giving sight to the blind is now
more often feasible. We already live in an age of miracles, in which sight
is being restored by such unanticipated methods as using part of someone's
tooth to enable sight or using gene therapy or even nanotechnology. But
in our excitement at the prospect of restoring a person's sight we failed to
understand that the mechanics of restoring visual input to the brain—to
the visual cortex—is not the same thing as restoring seeing.

For instance, in 2000 skier Michael May had his sight fully restored
after having been blind since he was three and a half years old. May underwent a cornea transplant and a groundbreaking new stem cell procedure that enabled doctors to cure his blindness. But even two years after
he had his sight restored he was still living in a world where he could make
no sense of visual patterns. After some years of therapy he still could not
recognize his wife by looking at her face or looking at a photograph of her,
but he could instantly recognize her by touching her face. Similarly, he
found it easier to ski before he regained his sight than after he regained it.
The movie *At First Sight*, staring Val Kilmer, is based on various reports
by Oliver Sachs of patients recovering their sight after many years of
being blind. This movie, too, portrays someone who has far greater difficulty coming to terms with regaining his sight than he thought he would
have.

The age at which people lose their sight, or whether they ever had
sight, is a significant factor in what they will experience should the physical mechanics of sight be restored to them, whether by medical means or
by accident. If a person is born blind, or if he or she loses sight at a very
young age, then the brain will not have learned *how* to see. As normally
sighted people, we take this for granted; of course we know what seeing
is, and of course every blind person would want to have sight if the option were available. But the reality is that if the brain has not created the
neural pathways and connections associated with seeing and processing
visual information—making sense of visual data—then the mere act of
reconnecting visual input to the brain will not mean the person can suddenly see.

Reports on this are quite consistent: the greater the time between loss
of sight and regaining it, then the greater the difficulty the person has seeing, once sight is restored. If the person was born blind or lost his or her
sight at a very young age, then as our science currently stands, restoration
of sight is unlikely, even if a technique restores visual data to the brain

or if an artificial device is implanted that feeds visual data into the brain, much as a normally functioning human eye does.

This relates to the common misconception that blind people are somehow less whole than those of us who have all five senses. We jump to the conclusion that if blind people have their sight restored to them, they will become whole again if they had lost their sight, or become whole for the first time if they never had it. But the reality is that, for blind people, restoring their sight is not like throwing a light switch in a darkened room, whereupon they can suddenly see everything exactly as sighted people can see everything. This can be very puzzling for the friends and loved ones of a blind person contemplating having an operation to restore sight. Why would blind people have any hesitancy over regaining their sight? Why would they not want to become whole again? Why would they not want to see what you or their children or their family or their friends look like?

At the end of several decades of active research into restoring sight, science finds itself at the beginning of a journey, then, not at the end of it. Now we appreciate that beyond restoring the basic mechanics of seeing—switching back on the capability for visual data to be sent to the brain—we now need to explore ways to help the previously blind person make sense of the visual data, once it is restored. And what we are fast learning is that this process is far from simple. There is a common misconception shared even within the scientific community, that it is nearly impossible to teach a mature brain how to process information that it did not learn how to process in the first few years of life. On the contrary, while there is some basic truth to the brain's being far more plastic in the early years, the human brain also never fails to amaze in its ability to adapt. Often when people lose a faculty later in life—say, through brain damage—other parts of the brain take over and adapt to process the information instead of the damaged part of the brain.

For instance, the potential exists for a next generation of technology that could perhaps assist in cross-modal sensory training or cross-sensory mapping: rather than merely feeding raw visual data to the visual cortex, technology could feed the data from the recovered eye or the device to both the visual and sensory cortices so that seeing an object could be cross-trained with the sense of touching it. The device could, for instance, not only detect that the previously blind person is looking at a face (we have had accurate face-perception technology for some time now) but also sense that the person is touching the face at the same time and synthesize the data so that, in future, looking at that same face would invoke a ghost sensation of touching it. In this way, the new sense data (visual input) could be cross-trained with familiar data (the sense of touch from hands on a person's face), enabling the mature brain to convert the un-familiar visual data into a form it could more easily process. While this may sound farfetched, it or some other approach that seeks to map the new sensory modality with an existing known modality may prove to be a fruitful line of research. Certainly, with these anticipated techniques and technologies, a previously blind person would not learn to see in the same sense that a normally sighted person sees (a person whose brain has had decades to learn how to process visual data in order to see); but the previ-ously blind person would be able to develop a new sense, a new modality, that would at least parallel what normally sighted people call *seeing*.

How else could such a cross-modal mapping help the previously blind, once the mechanics of seeing have been restored? Well, for instance, a key challenge blind people face is knowing where objects are in a room. To cope, the blind will have mapped out any familiar space (say, their of-fice or home) and learned where every piece of furniture is, every door-way, and so on. They will have counted the steps from one location to the next. Needless to say, they cannot adopt these strategies in a new envi-ronment that they have not yet learned. But if devices and accompany-ing training techniques could be devised whereby previously blind people could effectively "feel at a distance"—by looking at something and having the device evoke the sense of touch generated by that object—then they could effectively "see" furniture in a room that they have never been in before, because while they might have difficulty seeing a table as a table in the sense normally sighted people see it, they could sense an object that is linked to the touch sensation they associate with a table. Is this far-fetched? Not really, for in a way such techniques and devices would paral-lel the way that bats see using sonar. While not yet a scientific reality at the time of writing, such devices and techniques may well be the way that blind people are given a new sense of sight in the future, one that is both more than and less than what regularly sighted people call sight.

But is that true? Wouldn't this synthesized sight always be less than *real* natural sight? On the contrary, just like amputees who have won awards for running with prosthetic legs, the technologically enhanced resighted person could have abilities regularly sighted people lack. Aside from an ability to combine different sensory perceptions, there is the basic act of sight itself: sight depends on what visual wavelengths of light are avail-able: quite simply, the range of light from red to violet constitutes the fre-quencies of light our eyes are attuned to process. But no such limitations will exist for artificially sighted persons. There is no reason, for instance, why in restoring sight using a device other than the human eye, it would not be possible to add the ability to see in the infrared and ultraviolet ends of the spectrum. It may sound as though this is at the boundaries of science fact and science fiction, but someone capable of seeing in the infrared end of the spectrum would be able to see, for example, whether a pot on a stove was too hot to touch well before being close enough to sense the heat radiating from it. This person would also, to some extent, be able to see through walls, since heat radiation passes through walls whereas light in the visual spectrum does not. But would someone with artificial sight want such enhancements? That would surely be a matter of individual preference, but since those with the option for prosthetics, having lost limbs, have chosen technology that would enable them to do more than they could have done with the limbs they lost, it is highly likely that those seeking to gain artificial sight will indeed opt for abilities regularly sighted people lack.

That isn't to say that gaining such supersight would be without its pitfalls and problems. For instance, consider the idea of seeing in the infrared part of the spectrum. It might enable the person to see through walls effectively if there was anything (or anyone) on the other side giving off heat, but what if the ability could not be switched off? Would one want to be able to see people through walls at all times? Probably not, given that such an ability would enable the supersighted person to see people inside restrooms and inside private rooms where the other person may have gone specifically not to be seen. Like most scientific advances, supersight will come with pros and cons. It is already possible to purchase infrared binoculars like those used by spies and the military, thus those who might abuse such supersight already have the means to do so.

## WHAT IS SEEING?

This may seem like a nonsensical question—surely we all know what seeing is? Actually, that is far from the truth and is a topic that could easily fill a separate book. Suffice it to say, there is no objective visual world that each of us sees in the sense that objects exist separate from our concepts of them or in which we all see the same objects, the same colors, and so forth. Decades of scientific research and literally hundreds of years of philosophy have taught us that the brain works somewhat like a hypothesis engine that speculates about what it is seeing and makes its best guess. Consider, for instance, the room around you. Assuming it has colored walls, paintings on the walls, or perhaps wallpaper, do you see yourself in a fully colored room? Most likely you do. And yet at the periphery of your vision you can see only movement and black and white images; you cannot see color outside the central area of your vision. Why then do you perceive the colored walls, the wallpaper, the colored paintings, and so on, as color even in your periphery? It is because the brain fills in the information it does not have with what it believes it knows from prior experience and successful hypothesis. This also explains why, late at night in the shadows, you might be quite certain you saw a dog move, only to discover it was just the wind stirring up leaves. But for a moment you actually "saw" a dog and could perhaps even describe the breed and coloration of the dog. The mind is a powerful generator of illusions, especially visual ones.

Another example of how the brain hypothesizes is the way we perceive distance. Just as the timing of sounds reaching our ears and the phase difference in the sound waves hitting each outer ear enable us to tell where in three-dimensional space a sound emanates from, so the fact that our eyes are a few inches apart enables us to see depth. But as someone with only one eye—particularly someone born with only one eye—will tell us, the idea of depth is based on numerous calculations the brain makes and not a given truth that all people perceive. Indeed, the mind can be tricked quite easily by having an object that is larger than you usually expect it to be set nearer than another object that is smaller than you usually expect it to be. At first, your mind will perceive the larger object as being closer, even if it is not, simply because of what you are used to perceiving. The brain makes calculations based on what it thinks it knows, not on some absolute fact about the raw visual data it is receiving.

All this only goes to underscore the immense challenge facing previously blind persons who have sight restored, particularly if they have lost the ability of *how* to see or if they were born blind. It is not simply a matter of (re)learning what a door looks like, what a table looks like, or what a face looks like (let alone a specific door, table, or face) but a matter of learning or relearning complex concepts that for normally sighted persons took years to develop fully, and at a time when the brain was far more plastic than it is in a mature adult.

## SCIENTIFIC BREAKTHROUGHS

Finding aids or cures for visual impairment has, of course, been the goal of many people for well over a thousand years. As long ago as the 5th century B.C., Egyptian hieroglyphs depicted the use of concave and convex (so-called meniscus) lenses. And as long ago as the 1st century A.D., in the time of the Emperor Nero, the use of globes filled with water for viewing indistinct writing is reported, and Nero himself is reported to have used a polished emerald to see gladiator fights more clearly. It wasn't until the early 13th century, though, that Salvino D'Armate created what are thought to be the first wearable spectacles. Then, jumping forward to 1784, Benjamin Franklin invented the first bifocal lenses to correct for both shortsightedness and farsightedness.

Perhaps even more surprising, though, is how long ago the first cataract treatments occurred. In the sixth century B.C. the Indian physician Sushruta wrote the *Sushruta Samhita* (Bhishagratna), in which he describes a technique called *couching* that he claimed could cure cataracts. This method continued to be used well into the Middle Ages, although it was usually dangerous and could easily leave the patient completely blind. The first successful cataract treatment in Europe was by Jacques Daviel in 1748, and then more recently in the 1940s Harold Riley developed a technique that used a foldable intraocular lens, which made the procedure more comfortable and recovery quicker. Then in 1967 Charles Kelman invented a technique called phacoemulsification, which makes modern cataract removal relatively painless and recovery very swift.

But despite the many centuries of work on using lenses of one kind or another to correct for deficiencies in sight, and a long history of removing cataracts, it is only in the past decade or so that significant advances have been made in curing blindness or aiding those with deficient sight outside of the use of lenses and cataract removal. It seems that now no year goes by without a news story announcing "Surgeons Hail Blindness Cure," "Blind Woman Sees with Tooth Implanted in Eye Surgery," "Bionic Eye Unveiled," "Gene Cure to Blindness," or "Stem Cell Contact Lenses Cure Blindness in Less Than a Month."

Our goal here is not to provide an exhaustive survey of all the work done recently on curing blindness but rather to give a general overview of just some of the key research. What is readily apparent is the incredible diversity of approaches being explored, together with greater probability than ever before that blindness previously thought to be incurable may actually be curable.

Before moving on to technological advances, though, let's consider some of the more random events that have led to improvement in sight. For instance, Malcolm Darby, a 70-year-old from the county of Leicestershire in England, had a stroke 2009 and almost fully recovered his sight despite being close to legally blind since the age of 2. He experienced the stroke and was rushed to a hospital, where he had a blood clot removed. Suddenly, upon waking from surgery, he realized he could read the headlines of newspapers across the room—something he had never been able to do before. There is no clear explanation for Darby's recovery of sight, but there was an odd side effect: prior to his stroke he was fluent in French, whereas afterward he was unable to speak a single word of French. If nothing else, as Ellen Branagh observes, this incident highlights the mysterious way the brain works and ultimately how little we still know about the brain (Branagh).

And Darby is not the only person to recover sight after a stroke. In 2006, 74-year-old Joyce Urch, also in England, awoke in the hospital after a heart attack to find she could see again after being completely blind for the prior 25 years. When she came round from her operation her first words were "I can see! I can see!" Turning to her husband, she said, "You've got older, haven't you?" She was now able to see her five children for the first time since they were young adults and able to see her 12 grandchildren and 3 great-grandchildren for the first time. Over the 25 years she had had numerous treatments, none of which enabled her to see again. But as a result of the heart attack she was able to see again immediately, and nearly perfectly. Urch had been suffering from glaucoma, but for years doctors did not believe that it was the source of her blindness. Indeed, they remained puzzled by her loss of sight and had come to believe it might be a genetic disorder. The reason for her full cure from blindness remains a mystery to this day (Britten).

To be clear, no one is advocating having a heart attack as a remedy for blindness. Indeed, needless to say, many blind people suffer heart attacks and do not recover their sight. But what is clear is that there is in some cases a connection between brain function and sight that remains a mystery. Eventually, scientists will be able to unravel what took place in people like Darby and Urch and be able to simulate it in the brain so as to induce recovery of sight in others in safe, controlled conditions.

Perhaps one of the more bizarre-sounding, yet consistently successful, treatments for blindness involves a tooth transplant. As Britain's newspaper *The Daily Telegraph* ("Blind Man...") reported in July 2009, a 42-year-old builder, Martin Jones, who had been blind for 12 years, recovered his sight through a revolutionary new technique involving implanting one of his teeth into his eye. A factory accident in which white hot aluminum exploded in his face left him without his left eye, and while his right eye was saved he was unable to see with it. The technique modified his tooth into a lens holder, thereby enabling him to see again. And within hours after recovering from the surgery, Jones was able to see his wife of four years for the very first time. The procedure was carried out in Brighton, England, by Christopher Lui, the only specialist at the time capable of doing the operation. Lui was also the president of the British Society for Refractive Surgery.

This amazing procedure, which left Jones looking like a character from a sci-fi movie, involved extracting one of his canine teeth and using it to hold a constructed lens. The canine tooth was selected as the best suited to hold a lens due to its size and shape. A tooth was used because there would be a far higher chance of the body rejecting a plastic equivalent. A patch of skin was taken from inside Jones's cheek and implanted in his right eyelid for two months while it acquired its own blood supply. The tooth was then transplanted into the eye and the flap of skin from his inner cheek grafted over the end. Finally, the surgeons cut a hole in the grafted cornea to let the light through. The technique was developed to help patients who needed corneal transplants but who were not well suited for traditional transplant procedures. Said Jones in a newspaper interview at the time, "Getting my sight back has changed my life. It is such a precious gift, and you don't really appreciate it until it is taken away" (*Daily Telegraph*).

More recently, in September 2009, ABC News reported the first U.S. surgery took place to enable a woman to recover her sight by the same tooth implant procedure (technically called modified osteo-odonto-keratoprosthesis, or MOOKP) ("Blind woman..."). Doctors in Miami were able to restore 60-year-old Kay Thornton's sight from complete blindness to 20/70 vision. As with Martin Jones in Britain, she had one of her teeth removed and transplanted into her eye. A hole was drilled in the tooth to enable it to house a small plastic lens as a replacement cornea. Thornton had been blind for nine years, having lost her sight owing to Stevens-Johnson syndrome. As with Jones, previous attempts to use gene therapy to cure her condition had not been successful, but with the MOOKP procedure, she was able to see as soon as the bandages were removed from her face.

Thornton had been feeling very challenged by her blindness. In an interview with CNN she said, "It was very embarrassing and humiliating [to me] for my daughter to take care of me, and it wasn't supposed to be that way. I'm supposed to take care of her. I thought about suicide, but then I thought, if I did it, I probably wouldn't do it right. I just asked God to help me. I couldn't do it by myself. He taught me patience, and I never gave up" ("Blind woman...").

Currently, MOOKP is rarely used and usually only in circumstances in which there is insufficient moisture on the surface of the eye to permit a more usual corneal transplant to take place. Indeed, the procedure was inspired by doctors in Asia and Europe noting the similarity between moisture in the mouth and in the eye ("Blind woman..."). True inspiration indeed.

In March 2008, news stories hailed a drug to cure blindness as a "break-through," and as a result scientists were predicting a complete cure to blindness would occur within five years. To be more specific, the cure is for macular degeneration, previously thought to cause irreversible blindness in millions of people every year. Indeed, macular degeneration is the leading cause of blindness in people 65 or older, thus making this drug cure particularly noteworthy. Kang Zhang (Jones), then at the University of Utah School of Medicine, was coauthor of a study in the journal *Nature Medicine* that reported that blindness can be reversed by injecting drugs that activate a protein known as Robo4 in blood vessel cells. Zhang reported that use of these drugs could dramatically increase the chances of patients suffering from macular degeneration or diabetic retinopathy of recovering their sight. Dean Li, senior author of the study, announced (Jones) that in his opinion the technique could start being used to cure patients within five years, and according to recent reports his predication seems on schedule.

In April 2010, scientists reported that a new gene therapy had been successful in restoring sight to blind dogs and that such techniques could soon be used on human patients. The particular cause of blindness in this case is congenital achromatopsia, also called rod monochromacy, or total color blindness. Achromatopsia is rare in humans, occurring in as few as 1 in 30,000 to 50,000 people, but therapy for the disease had been relatively unheard of prior to this discovery. The gene therapy is targeted at variations of the CNGB3 gene, which is a common cause of achromatopsia in humans. "The successful restoration of visual function with recombinant adeno-associated virus-mediated gene replacement therapy has ushered in a new era of retinal therapeutics," said András M. Komáromy, assistant professor of Ophthalmology at the Penn School of Veterinary Medicine and lead author of the study. (RedOrbit)

Stem cell research has also provided procedures for curing blindness. In August 2009, researchers from the University of Florida claimed to be the first to use targeted gene manipulation to change adult stem cells into a totally different type of cell (Chun). Using their technique they were able to change bone marrow cells into retinal cells, which cured blindness when injected into blind mice. Most important, these techniques used adult cells, not embryonic stem cells, thus providing hope for alternatives to the more controversial embryonic stem cell research.

Gene therapy is helping to cure various forms of blindness. In March 2010, scientists from Buffalo, Cleveland, and Oklahoma City broke new ground when they used gene therapy to cure blindness without modifing viruses. They were seeking a cure for blindness associated with retinitis pigmentosa and other acquired and inherited retinal diseases. Muna Naash, a researcher from the Department of Cell Biology at the University of Oklahoma Heath Sciences Center in Oklahoma City, reported, "Compacted DNA nanoparticles are an exciting treatment strategy for these diseases, and we look forward to exciting new developments." Naash and colleagues worked with mice who had the gene known to cause retinitis pigmentosa known as the retinal degeneration slow (Rds) gene. The mice were given nanoparticles containing a normal copy of the Rds gene and to recovered their sight. "Making the blind see was once called a miracle," said Gerald Weissmann, editor in chief of the *FASEB Journal*. "As we have expanded our understanding of evolution, genetics, and nanotechnology, chances are that "miraculous" cures will become as commonplace as those claimed by faith-healers past and present" (Physorg).

Last but not least, there is the extensive research going on to create bionic eyes to replace sight. For the past 20 years, scientists at the Boston Retinal Implant Project (Boston Retinal Implant Project) have been developing a bionic implant that could restore sight to people with age-related blindness. The implant uses state-of-the-art miniaturized electronics and involves a chip being implanted behind the retina at the back of the eyeball. An ultrathin wire strengthens the damaged optic nerve, and the wire transmits light and images directly to the visual cortex, where the brain can process the signals normally as if being sent from a real human eye. The rest of the device sits outside the eye and would most likely be mounted in spectacle frames.

More recently, in April 2010, Bionic Vision Australia (BVA) announced a new neurostimulator project—a bionic eye that they are implanting in a blind human patient ("Bionic Eye...")e. Like the Boston project, BVA's device involves a miniature camera mounted on spectacles to capture visual input, which is then transformed into electronic signals that directly stimulate the remaining surviving neurons in the retina. Even if full sight cannot be recovered, the researchers believe that the brain will be able to construct sufficient information from points of light delivered by the device to enable to recipient to have significantly increased mobility and independence. As with other techniques, the BVA device is particularly targeted at age-related blindness like retinitis pigmentosa and retinal degeneration.

Interestingly, the scientists in the Boston research study underscore the fact that this technique will be useful only for recovering sight in patients who once had sight since the brain must already know how to process visual information for this bionic eye to work. This, of course, takes us full circle to the earlier discussion of this issue: that the physical restoration of sight does not ensure that a patient will be able to see again as a normally sighted person can. Much will depend on whether the person could see before and how long he or she has been blind. But as we discussed above, even in extreme cases, in which someone has been blind since birth or has lost his or her sight at a very young age, there are still innovative techniques waiting to be devised, like the cross-modal approach we have proposed in this book, that may enable a new form of sight to be gained by previously blind people. Certainly, it will not be sight in exactly the same sense as for the normally sighted person, but it will be sight nonetheless. And as the cases of spontaneous recovery from blindness have taught us, we should never underestimate the brain's ability to adapt and recover. Even in adulthood, beyond the early years, clearly the brain is still capable of adapting.

Although it may sound like science fiction today, at some point we may be able to train the brain to grow a new visual cortex and establish many of the same functions as are in a normally sighted person, even down to the brain being accelerated in learning how to interpret visual imagery. If the astounding recent research on curing blindness has taught us anything, it is that there is tremendous hope for new cures that at this time we cannot even begin to imagine.

# 7

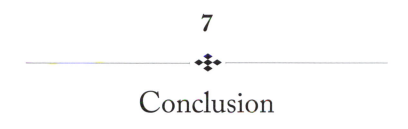

# Conclusion

The only thing worse than being blind is having sight but no vision.

Helen Keller

Vision loss does not have to be detrimental but can actually be empowering. It is all in your attitude. Technologically speaking, there has never been a greater array of devices available for the visually impaired or greater hope of technological and medical solutions for curing blindness and aiding the visually impaired in new ways. So much can be done through the Internet and e-mail, through using speaking computers and talking books, that the world of sighted people is fast becoming more and more accessible to the visually impaired. No longer does a diagnosis of blindness need to carry with it the stigma of isolation from society in general. There are talking ATM machines for banking, appliances are becoming more accessible, many communities have paratransit to provide inexpensive transportation, and there are other services. Medically speaking, there is so much on the horizon: support groups and e-mail lists are abundant. Rehabilitation and education are there for the asking in most communities and worldwide via the Internet.

As we have seen in this book, going blind need not be the curse it was once thought to be. Not only do we have an abundance of blind people living full rich lives and achieving greatness and fame in various fields but we also have an ever growing probability that most, and perhaps all, forms of blindness may become curable within our lifetimes. Conditions we believed were completely irreversible and incurable just 10 to 15 years ago are either now curable or we can at least see significant scientific progress toward curing them. We expect the next decade will bring still more progress for those who are visually challenged, so we advocate maintaining an openness to new scientific research since groundbreaking research has already restored the sight of many, and as we saw in the last chapter, it is never too late and one is never too old to regain one's sight.

# Appendix

❖

# List of Useful Links and Resources

American Action Fund for Blind Children and Adults, provide blind services beyond government and other programs. http://www.actionfund.org/actionfund/Default.asp

American Council of the Blind, "fulfilling Helen Keller's vision." The American Council of the Blind describes itself as "the nation's leading membership organization of blind and visually impaired people. ACB. . . has 51 state and regional affiliates and 20 national special interest and professional affiliates" and has "tens of thousands of members." Finally, "The Council strives to improve the well-being of all blind and visually impaired people by: serving as a representative national organization of blind people; elevating the social, economic and cultural levels of blind people; improving educational and rehabilitation facilities and opportunities; cooperating with the public and private institutions and organizations concerned with blind services; encouraging and assisting all blind persons to develop their abilities and conducting a public education program to promote greater understanding of blindness and the capabilities of blind people." The Braille Forum is a free national magazine published by the ACB. http://www.acb.org/

American Foundation for the Blind styles itself as "a US nonprofit organization enabling blind or visually impaired people to achieve equality and access." http://www.afb.org/

American Printing House for the Blind, source for adapted educational and daily living products. http://www.aph.org/

Apple Resources, products for the blind and visually impaired. http://www.apple.com/accessibility/

Assemblies of God National Center for the Blind, Assistive Technology Center, bridging adaptive and mainstream technologies. http://blind.ag.org/

Beyond Sight, products for the blind and visually impaired. http://www.beyondsight.com/

Bibles for the Blind and Visually Handicapped, Bibles in different media, plus links to helpful resources. http://www.biblesfortheblind.org/

BlindCoolTech, fun, educational podcasts for MP3 players. http://blindcooltech.com/

Blinded Veterans Association, promoting the welfare of blinded veterans. http://www.bva.org/

Braille Bug, Web site for blind and visually impaired children. http://www.afb.org/braillebug/

Braille Collection, jewelry with a Braille theme. http://www.braille jewelry.com/

Braille Institute of America, affording hope and encouragement for people who are blind. http://www.brailleinstitute.org/

Braille International Inc., enhancing the independence and quality of life for blind persons. http://www.brailleintl.org/

BRL: Braille through Remote Learning, learn Braille online. http://www.brl.org/

Callahan Museum of APH, collection of early mechanical Braille writers and other artifacts. http://www.aph.org/museum/

Canadian National Institute for the Blind. According to their Web site, they provide "services to people who are blind, visually impaired and deaf-blind in order to enhance their independence. The CNIB provides services at no cost to people of all ages. We have structured our organization to meet the needs of children under 18, working-age adults, and seniors, through our seven core services." They provide sight enhancement, counseling, orientation, help with mobility, and a wide range of other vital services. http://www.cnib.ca/

Chicago Lighthouse, for people who are blind or visually impaired. http://chicagolighthouse.org/

Clovernook Center, for the blind and visually impaired. http://www.clovernook.org/

Descriptive Video Service, making television and movies more accessible to people who are blind or have low vision. http://main.wgbh.org/wgbh/pages/mag/services/description/

*Diabetes Forecast*, a magazine published by the American Diabetes Association. http://forecast.diabetes.org/

Disability Digest, a free daily e-mail newsletter for the blind and those with disabilities. The focus is on helping the visually challenged American get access to the benefits he or she is entitled to. http://www.the disabilitydigest.com

Dotless Braille, a new approach to Braille. http://www.dotlessbraille.org/

Duxbury Systems, a multiplatform, multilanguage Braille translator. http://www.duxburysystems.com/

Family friendly fun and special needs resources. http://www.family-friendly-fun.com/

Fred's Head Database, tips and techniques for the blind and visually impaired. http://www.aph.org/fh/index.html

Freedom Scientific, provider of reading systems for people with visual and reading disabilities. http://www.freedomscientific.com/

GW Micro, independence to the visually impaired through computer-based speech products. http://www.synapseadaptive.com/gw/gwhome. htm

Hebrew Visions, helping blind individuals gain access to digital texts in Hebrew Braille. http://www.hebrewvisions.org/

Humanware. http://www.humanware.com/en-usa/home

IntelliTools, technology for learning. http://www.intellitools.com/

Jewish Braille Institute International. http://www.jewishvirtuallibrary. org/jsource/Orgs/jbi.html

Kurzweil Educational Systems. http://www.kurzweiledu.com/

Labels for Literacy, equal access to information. http://www.labelsforlit eracy.org/

LevelStar. http://www.levelstar.com/

Louis Braille School, an academic program for blind children. http://louisbrailleschool.org/

Lutheran Blind Mission, a Christian outreach with the visually impaired. http://www.blindmission.org/

Lutheran Braille Workers. http://www.lbwinc.org/

Matilda Ziegler Magazine for the Blind. http://www.matildaziegler.com/

MoPix, movie theater accessibility. http://ncam.wgbh.org/mopix/

National Association of the Visually Handicapped (now part of Lighthouse International). http://lighthouse.org/navh

National Braille Press, printing and publishing Braille since 1927. http://www.nbp.org/

National Federation of the Blind. http://www.nfb.org/

National Library Service for the Blind and Physically Handicapped. http://www.loc.gov/nls/

New York Institute for Special Education Blindness Resource Center. http://www.nyise.org/blind.htm

Online communities focusing on blindness at Yahoo! http://dir.groups.
  yahoo.com/dir/1600189052?st=10
Optelec, video magnifiers and low-vision aids. http://www.optelec.com/
  home
Perkins School for the Blind. http://www.perkins.org/
Royal National Institute for the Blind. http://www.rnib.org.uk/
Sendero Group, GPS for the blind. http://www.senderogroup.com/
TACK-TILES Braille Systems. http://www.tack-tiles.com/
TechAdapt. accessible media services. http://www.techadapt.com/

# Works Cited and Consulted

Alant, Erna and Lyle L. Lloyd, Eds. *Augmentative and Alternative Communication and Severe Disabilities, Beyond Poverty*. London: Whurr Publishers, 2005.

Al-Arabi, Ibn. *101 Diamonds, from the Oral Tradition of the Glorious Messenger Muhammad*. New York: Pir Press, 2002.

Appelbaum, Stanley (Ed). *Lazarillo de Tormes (Dual Language)*. Mineola, NY: Dover Publications, 2001.

Ar-Rifa'i as-Shadhuli, Shaykh Muhammad Sa'id al-Jamal. *Music of the Soul*. 3rd ed. Petaluma, CA: Sidi Muhammad Press, 2002.

Ar-Rifa'i as-Shadhuli, Shaykh Muhammad Sa'id al-Jamal. *The Ocean of the Mercy*. Petaluma, CA: Sidi Muhammad Press, 2005.

Ar-Rifa'i as-Shadhuli, Shaykh Muhammad Sa'id al-Jamal. *Stories of the Prophets*. Petaluma, CA: Sidi Muhammad Press, 1996.

*At First Sight*. Dir. Irwin Winkler. Perf. Val Kilmer, Mira Sorvino, and Kelly McGillis. Metro-Goldwyn-Meyer. 1999.

Atwood, Margaret. *Writing with Intent: Essays, Reviews, Personal Prose, 1983–2005*. New York: Carroll & Graf, 2005.

Bachman, Maria K. "'Furious Passions of the Celtic Race'": Ireland, Madness and Wilkie Collins's *Blind Love*." *Victorian Crime, Madness and Sensation*. Ed. Andrew Maunder and Grace Moore. Aldershot, UK: Ashgate, 2004. 179–194.

Ballin, Albert. *The Deaf Mute Howls*. Washington, DC: Gallaudet University Press, 1998.

Bauman, Mary K., and Norman H. Yoder. *Adjustment to Blindness—Reviewed*. Springfield, IL, 1966.

Bhalerad, Usha. *Blind Women's Emancipation Movement, A World Perspective*. New Delhi: Sterling, 1986.

Bhishagratna, Kaviraj Kunjalal. *The Sushruta Samihita: An English Translation Based on Original Texts*. New Delhi: Cosmo Publications, 2006.

"Bionic eye attempts to restore VISION." *Wired* Magazine Online. April 2, 2010. http://www.wired.com/gadgetlab/2010/04/australian-bionic-eye/.

"Blind man has sight restored by having tooth implanted in his eye." *The Daily Telegraph*, July 4, 2009. http://www.telegraph.co.uk/news/newstopics/howaboutthat/5737927/Blind-man-has-sight-restored-by-having-tooth-implanted-in-his-eye.html.

"Blind woman sees with 'tooth-in-eye' surgery." ABC News, September 17, 2009. http://abcnews.go.com/Health/Technology/woman-regains-vision-tooth-implanted-eye/story?id=8595589.

Boston Retinal Implant Project. http://www.bostonretinalimplant.org/.

Branagh, Ellen. "Man gains normal eyesight after stroke at 70." Sep. 2, 2009. http://www.independent.co.uk/life-style/health-and-families/health-news/man-gains-normal-eyesight-after-stroke-at-70–1780632.html.

Britten, Nick. "I had been blind 25 years. I had a heart attack, woke up, and could see. I said to my husband: 'You've got older.' " *Daily Telegraph*, Jan. 20, 2006. http://www.telegraph.co.uk/news/uknews/1508273/I-had-been-blind-25-years.-I-had-a-heart-attack-woke-up-and-could-see.-I-said-to-my-husband-Youve-got-older.html.

Carver, Raymond. "Cathedral." *Literature, Reading, Reacting, Writing*. Ed. Laurie Kirszner and Stephen Mandell. New York: Harcourt Brace College, 1997.

Cholden, Louis S. *A Psychiatrist Works with the Blind*. New York: American Foundation for the Blind, 1958.

Chun, Diane. "Sight gene therapy works wonders." *The Gainesville Sun*, Aug. 13, 2009. http://www.gainesville.com/article/20090813/ARTICLES/908131042.

Collins, Wilkie. *Poor Miss Finch*. New York: Harper, 1899.

Conway, Flo, and Jim Spiegelman. *Snapping: America's Epidemic of Sudden Personality Change*. 2nd Edition. New York: Stillpoint Press, 1995.

Cunningham, Caranda, and Norman Cousins. *Information Access and Adaptive Technology*. Phoenix: American Council of Education, Oryx Press, 1997.

*Deliverance*. Dir. George Foster Platt. Perf. Etna Ross and Ann Mason. Hellen Keller Film Corporation, 1919.

Derrida, Jacques. *Memoirs of the Blind: The Self-Portrait and Other Ruins*. Chicago: University of Chicago Press, 1993.

Dickinson, Emily. "I heard a Fly buzz—when I died" *The Poems of Emily Dickinson*, Vol. 2. R. W. Franklin, ed. Cambridge, MA: Belknap, 1998, 587.

Doyle, Richard E. *ATH: Its Use and Meaning*. New York: Fordham University Press, 1984.

Dunn, Phillip, Manuela Mascentti, and R.A. Nicholson. *The Illustrated Rumi*. New York: HarperOne, 2000.

Eckhart, Meister, from *Whom God Hid Nothing: Sermons, Writings, and Sayings*. David O'Neal, ed. Boston and London: New Seeds, 2005.

Eliot, George. *Middlemarch*. Oxford, UK: Oxford University Press, 1996.

Ellmann, Richard, and Robert O'Clair. *The Norton Anthology of Modern Poetry*. 2nd ed. New York: Norton, 1988.

Fiedler, Leslie. Freaks: Myths and Images of the Secret Self. New York: Simon & Schuster, 1978.

Freedman, Diane P., and Martha Stoddard Holmes, eds. *The Teacher's Body: Embodiment, Authority, and Identity in the Academy*. Albany: State University of New York Press, 2003.

Fukurai, Shiro. *How Can I Make What I Cannot See?* New York: Van Nostrand Reinhold, 1974.

Gibson, William. *The Miracle Worker (A Play)*. New York: Scribner, 2008.

Glover, Jon, and Jon Silken. *The Penguin Book of First World War Prose*. London: Viking, 1989.

Goldstein, Evan R. "To Choose or Not to Choose." *The Chronicle Review*. Mar. 14, 2010. http://www.rcgd.isr.umich.edu/news/kitayama_ChronicleReview_3.14.10.pdf (September 23, 2010).

Hannninen, Kenneth A. *Teaching the Visually Handicapped*. Columbus, OH: Charles E. Merrill, 1975.

Hardy, Thomas. "The Man He Killed." *Modern British Poetry*. Ed. Louis Untermeyer, New York: Harcourt, Brace and Howe, 1920; Bartleby.com, 1999. www.bartleby.com/103/, 31 May 2010.

Hull, John. On Sight and Insight: *A Journey into the World of Blindness*. Oxford, UK: One World, 2001.

Ingersoll, Earle G. *Margaret Atwood: Conversations*. Princeton: Ontario Review P, 1990.

Jones, Christopher A., Nyall R. London, Haoyu Chen, et al. 2008. "Robo4 stabilizes the vascular network by inhibiting pathologic angiogenesis and endothelial hyperpermeabilit." *Nature Medicine* 14, 448–453.

Kastein, Shulamith, Isabelle Spaulding and Battia Scharf. *Raising the Young Blind Child: A Guide for Parents and Educators*. New York: Human Sciences Press, 1980.

Keller, Helen. *Helen Keller's Journal*. London: Michael Joseph, 1938.

Keller, Helen. *Out of the Dark. Essays, Letters, and Addresses on Physical and Social Vision*. Garden City, NY: Doubleday, Page, & Co., 1913.

Keller, Helen. *Selected Writings*. Ed. Kim E. Nielsen. New York: New York University Press, 2005.

Keller, Helen. Teacher: *Anne Sullivan Macy, by Helen Keller*. Garden City, NY: Doubleday, 1955.

Keller, Helen. The World I Live In *by Helen Keller*. New York: The Century Co., 1908.

Keller, Helen. *The Story of My Life*. Ed. Roger Shattuck with Dorothy Herrmann. New York: Norton, 1995.

Kelman, James. *How Late It Was*. New York: Norton, 1994.

Kennedy, John M. *Drawing and the Blind: Pictures to Touch*. New Haven: Yale University Press, 1993.

Kipling, Rudyard. "At Twenty-Two." *The Realm of Fiction, 74 Short Stories*. Ed. James B. Hall and Elizabeth Hall. New York: McGraw Hill, 1977. 83–91.

Kipling, Rudyard. *Indian Tales*. New York: Tudor Publishing, 1899.

Knott, Frederick. *Wait Until Dark*. New York: Dramatists' Play Service, 1967.

Krents, Howard. "Darkness at Noon." *The Student Writer, Editor and Critic*. Ed. Barbara Fine Clouse. 7th ed. Boston: McGraw-Hill, 2008, 234–36.

Kumar, Amitava, ed. *World Bank Literature*. Minneapolis: University of Minneapolis Press, 2003.

Kuusisto, Joseph. *Planet of the Blind*. New York: Dial, 1998.

Lash, Joseph P. *Helen Keller and Teacher: The Story of Helen Keller and Anne Sullivan Macy*. New York: Delacourte, 1980.

Lawrence, D. H. "The Blind Man." *The Norton Introduction to Literature*. Ed. Jerome Beaty. New York: Norton, 1973.

Lebens, Judith. "The theology of the text," Presentation May 1, 2008. Class Handout for Biblical Studies 1010, (Studies for Candidates for the M.Div.), Church Divinity School of the Pacific, Berkeley, CA (unpublished personal copy).

Liberman, Jacob. *Take Off Your Glasses And See*. New York: Three Rivers Press, 1995.

Lowenfeld, Berthold, ed. *The Visually Handicapped Child in School*. New York: John Day, 1973.

Mehta, Ved. *All for Love*. New York: Thunder's Mouth Press/Nation Books, 2001.

Mehta, Ved. *Face to Face*. Hammondsworth, UK: Penguin, 1958.

Mehta, Ved. *The Ledge Between the Streams*. New York: Norton, 1984.

Mehta, Ved. *The Stolen Light*. New York: Norton, 1989.

Mehta, Ved. *Up at Oxford*. New York/London: Norton, 1993.

Mehta, Ved. *Vedi*. New York: Oxford University Press, 1982.

Michalko, Rod. "I've Got a Blind Prof': The Place of Blindness in the Academy." *The Teacher's Body*. Eds. Diane P. Freedman and Martha Stoddard Holmes. Albany: State University of New York Press, 2003, 69–81.

Mills, Anne E., ed. *Language Acquisition in the Blind Child: Normal and Deficit*. London: Croom-Hill, 1983.

Moore, Mary B. *Desiring Voices: Women Sonneteers and Petrarchism*. Carbondale: Southern Illinois University Press, 2000.

Napier, Grace D. *Marissa, Obstacle Illusions*. Mesa, AZ: Selah Publishing Group, 2002.

Nelson, Cary, and Stephen Watt. *Academic Keywords: A Devil's Dictionary for Higher Education*. New York: Routledge, 1999.

Physorg. "Making the blind see: Gene therapy restores vision in mice." Mar. 31, 2010. http://www.physorg.com/news189267167.html.

Pineda, Cecile. *Face*. New York: Viking Penguin, 1985.

Porchia, Antonio. *Voices*. Port Townsend, WA: Copper Canyon Press, 2003.

Quiller-Couch, Arthur Thomas. *The Oxford Book of English Verse, 1250–1900*. Oxford: Clarendon, 1919. Bartleby.com, 1999. http://www.bartleby.com/br/101.html, 1 May 2010.

Rabby, Ramy, and Diane Croft. *Take Charge: A Strategic Guide for Blind Job Seekers*. Boston: National Braille Press, 1989.

Research to Prevent Blindness. http://www.rpbusa.org/rpb/.

RedOrbit. "Gene Therapy Cures Canine Blindness." Apr. 21, 2010. http://www.redorbit.com/news/science/1853461/gene_therapy_cures_canine_blindness/index.html.

Jalaluddin, Rumi. *The Essential Rumi. New Expanded Edition*. Coleman Barks, trans. New York: HarperOne, 2004.

Jalaluddin, Rumi. *The Illustrated Rumi: A Treasury of Wisdom from the Poet of the Soul*. Philip Dunn, Manuela Dunn Mascetti and R. A. Nicholson, Trans. New York: HarperOne, 2000.

Rusalem, Herbert. *Coping with the Unseen Environment: An Introduction to the Vocational Rehabilitation of Blind Persons*. New York: Teachers College Press, 1972.

Saramago, José. *Blindness*. New York: Harcourt Brace, 1997.

Schneider, Meir. *Self-Healing, My Life and Vision*. London: Routledge & Kegan Paul, 1987.

Scott, Eileen P. *Your Visually Impaired Student: A Guide for Teachers*. Baltimore: University Park Press, 1982.

Striker, Henri-Jacques. *A History of Disability*. Ann Arbor: U of Michigan P, 1999.

*The Unconquered*. Dir. Nancy Hamilton, Perf. Katharine Cornell, Helen Keller, Polly Thompson. Albert Margolies (Dist.)

Warren, David H. *Blindness and Early Childhood Development*. New York: American Foundation for the Blind, 1977.

Webster, Alec, and Joao Roe. *Children with Visual Impairments: Social Interaction, Language and Learning*. London: Routledge, 1998.

Wells, H. G. "The Country of the Blind." *The Literature Network*. Oct. 18, 2009. http://www.online-literature.com/wellshg/3/.

Whitt, Jan, and John C. Inscoe. "Wise Blood." *The New Georgia Encyclopedia*. Oct. 3, 2009. http://www.georgiaencyclopedia.org/nge/Article.jsp?id=h-478.

Whyte. "Sweet Darkness." http://www.panhala.net/Archive/Sweet_Darkness.html (September 24, 2010).

World Health Organization. http://www.who.int/en/

Wright, Richard. *Native Son*. New York: Harper & Row, 1940.

Yamada, Koun. *The Gateless Gate: Classic Book of Zen Koans*. Somerville, MA: Wisdom Publications, 2004.

# Index

## About the Authors

**Cheri Colby Langdell, PhD,** attended Westridge School, Vassar College, and Boston University. At the University of Southern California she earned her MA and PhD, and earned a TESOL Certificate at the University of California, Los Angeles. She then taught at the University of California at Riverside and California State University, Chico. She later taught at the University of Nottingham, Leicester University, and the University of London, Queen Mary College, and Birkbeck College. She has also taught English at the University of California, Riverside, and taught blind students and students with special needs at Riverside Community College and U.S. International College. She is now an adjunct professor of English at National University, teaching graduate courses online. She has published a number of articles and reviews, and her earlier books include *W. S. Merwin* (under her former name of Cheri Davis), and *Adrienne Rich: The Moment of Change.* Langdell has been keenly interested in working with and helping the blind since 2004, when she met Ann Morris Bliss and began to have a strong interest in helping the blind and both those who are coping with vision loss and those who are regaining their sight. Cheri and her husband Tim Langdell then became deeply engaged in investigating research under way on blindness, the psychology and literature of blindness, and contemporary cures for blindness.

**Tim Langdell, PhD,** attended Britain's Leicester University where he earned his BS jointly in physics and psychology. He then went on to

Nottingham University where he earned his MA in psychology, and then to University College, London, where he earned his PhD in clinical psychology. He trained at London's Institute of Psychiatry and the Maudsley Hospital, where he was a research psychologist, and he went on to teach at various UK universities. More recently, he has taught at the University of Southern California, and he is currently an associate professor in the Department of Media at National University, where he was chair and co-chair of the department. He is both a psychologist and a digital media expert. This is his fifth book.